THE SHRED
POWER
CLEANSE

ALSO BY IAN K. SMITH, M.D.

The SHRED Diet Cookbook

SUPER SHRED

SHRED

The Truth About Men

Eat

Happy

The 4 Day Diet

Extreme Fat Smash Diet

The Fat Smash Diet

The Take-Control Diet

Dr. Ian Smith's Guide to Medical Websites

The Blackbird Papers: A Novel

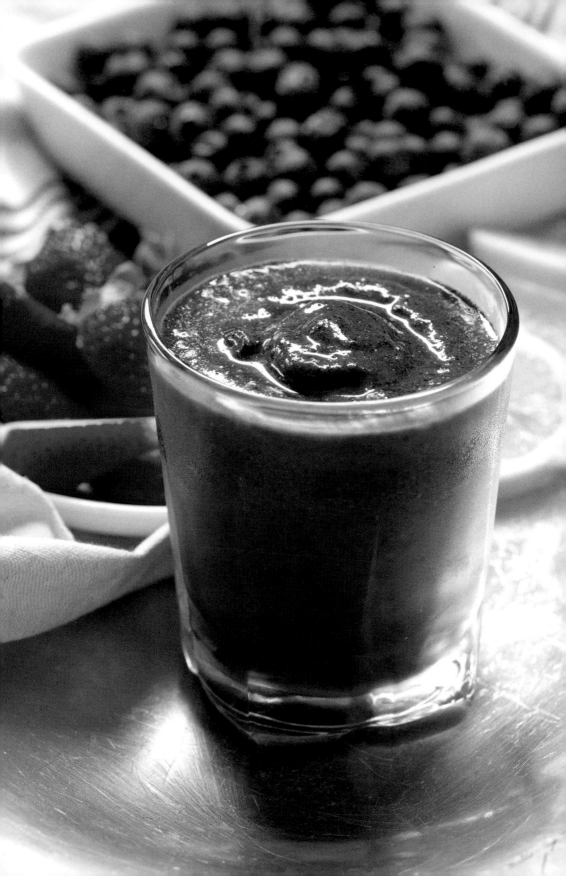

THE SHRED
POWER
CLEANSE

Eat Clean. Get Lean.
Burn Fat.

IAN K. SMITH, M.D.

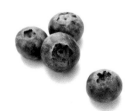

ST. MARTIN'S PRESS

New York

Note: This book is for informational purposes only. The author
has endeavored to make sure it contains reliable and accurate
information. However, research on diet and nutrition is evolving
and subject to interpretation, and the conclusions presented here
may differ from those found in other sources. As each individual's
experience may vary, readers, especially those with existing
health problems, should consult their physician or health-care
professional before adopting any nutritional changes based on
information contained in this book. Individual readers are solely
responsible for their own health-care decisions, and the author
and the publisher do not accept responsibility for any adverse
effects individuals may claim to experience, whether directly or
indirectly, based on information contained herein.

THE SHRED POWER CLEANSE.
Copyright © 2015 by Ian K. Smith, M.D.
All rights reserved. Printed in the United States of America.
For information, address St. Martin's Press, 175 Fifth Avenue,
New York, N.Y. 10010.

www.stmartins.com

The Library of Congress Cataloging-in-Publication Data is
available upon request.

ISBN 978-1-250-06122-5 (hardcover)
ISBN 978-1-4668-6686-7 (e-book)

Our books may be purchased in bulk for promotional,
educational, or business use. Please contact your local
bookseller or the Macmillan Corporate and Premium Sales
Department at 1-800-221-7945, extension 5442, or by e-mail at
MacmillanSpecialMarkets@macmillan.com.

First Edition: December 2015

10 9 8 7 6 5 4 3 2 1

To Tristé, Dashiell, and Declan. On a daily basis my sun rises and sets on you. I am intoxicated by the happiness you deliver. I love you forever.

CONTENTS

ACKNOWLEDGMENTS

To all who have come before me and sacrificed without complaint and whose shoulders I constantly stand on, I honor all that you have done and thank you for making it possible that I can continue to do what I love.

—

INTRODUCTION

We've all had times in our life when we've felt like we've splurged too hard on "fun foods" or that our bodies are sluggish from lack of movement and poor eating choices. The cliché "You are what you eat" is more than just a string of words. It's a great truth, and I would augment it to include, "You are how you move." The focus is on how we treat our bodies, amazing machines that operate best when given optimal fuel. This fuel doesn't have to be fancy or complicated. It doesn't have to be hard to find or only available to a certain segment of the population. This fuel is widely available, accessible, and easy to prepare so that you reap immediate benefits. The next fourteen days of the SHRED Power Cleanse will be dedicated to giving you what you need to feel better, look better, increase your energy, and fight disease in the most natural way possible—through clean food and efficient physical movement.

Toxin is a broad term to define chemicals or compounds that we ingest or inhale, actually unintentionally create inside of our bodies as a result of normal physiologic functioning. The body has an enormous ability to neutralize and eliminate toxins, which is important because these molecules can cause serious harm if they are left to accumulate. While the body goes through a detoxification process every second of every day, it also could be beneficial to enhance these functions through what is popularly called a *cleanse* or *detox*.

Cleanses and detox programs have been all the rage the last several years, with countless programs making at times unbelievable claims. But the fervor behind many of these cleanses is real. People want a chance to hit the reset button and start fresh. I have long been suspicious of these types of programs because I've believed that, while the intentions of the users are legitimate, many of the plans themselves tend to be unhealthy, whether overly restricting calorie intake or not providing sufficient nutrition.

Then I started to do research and began wondering if it were possible to use nature's power to help the body do something it already does very well—keep our systems clean and toxin-free. Was there a way to still take in enough calories and phytonutrients so our bodies aren't deprived—and at the same time aren't exposed to all the toxic chemicals we're typically not aware of in processed foods? Food in its most natural state has the same healing ability as medicine but without side effects. There's an enormous body of science that addresses how food can prevent and treat disease.

I then took a look at some startling statistics from the U.S. Centers for Disease Control and Prevention:

- **67 million** American adults (31 percent) have high blood pressure—that's **1 in every 3 adults.**
- About **1 in every 3 American adults** has **prehypertension**—blood pressure numbers that are higher than normal but not yet in the high blood pressure range.
- Only **about half (47 percent)** of people with high blood pressure have their condition under control.
- People with high cholesterol have about **twice the risk** of heart disease as people with lower levels.

Cholesterol is a waxy, fat-like substance. Your body needs some cholesterol, but it can build up on the walls of your arteries and lead to heart disease and stroke when you have too much in your blood.

- **71 million American adults (33.5 percent)** have high low-density lipoprotein (LDL), or bad, cholesterol.
- Only **1 in every 3** adults with high LDL cholesterol has the condition under control.
- **Less than half** of adults with high LDL cholesterol get treatment.

Lowering your cholesterol can reduce your risk of having a heart attack, needing heart bypass surgery or angioplasty, and dying of heart disease.

These statistics were only part of the story. The fact that medicines to treat these conditions are so widely available, yet the number of afflicted seems to be growing rather than diminishing, highlights the fact that all of our answers are not in a magic prescription bottle. There are natural and decisive food choices we can make today that can make a major contribution to overall wellness. Research consistently shows that these food choices should center on raw fruits, vegetables, whole grains, and herbaceous plants.

Armed with the knowledge that has long been attributed to Hippocrates, the father of modern medicine, "Let food be thy medicine," I decided to create a cleanse program that focused on going back to eating and drinking foods that are natural healers and health promoters. While it can take years to develop bad habits, the good news is that it doesn't take an enormous amount of time to recover and reverse some of the damage that has been done. In just 14 days, your life can be changed forever if you continue some of the healthy eating habits learned in this cleanse. I tested segments of the SHRED Power Cleanse with people from around the country, and the results were nothing short of amazing. Not only did people lose up to 10 pounds in two weeks, but they discovered that their blood pressure was lower and their cholesterol levels began to return to normal. In fact, some people no longer needed medications for these conditions, which they thought would afflict them for the rest of their lives.

This two-week program consists of nutrient-rich smoothies and shakes, along with one solid meal option per day. More than fifty recipes that can be used for the next two weeks are included with the program, as well as suggested exercises. This program uses some of the basic principles of the bestselling *SHRED* and *Super SHRED* diets, along with research from the National Heart, Blood, and Lung Institute that demonstrates foods and strategies scientifically proven to help lower blood pressure, as well as cholesterol conditions that affect over 140 million Americans and contribute to heart disease, the world's number 1 killer. In just two weeks, you can lose weight, lower your blood pressure, lower your cholesterol levels, feel GREAT, and not break the bank while doing it!

Move over green smoothie. The Purple Smoothie is now taking center stage.

Ian K. Smith, M.D.
Fall 2015

THE SHRED
POWER
CLEANSE

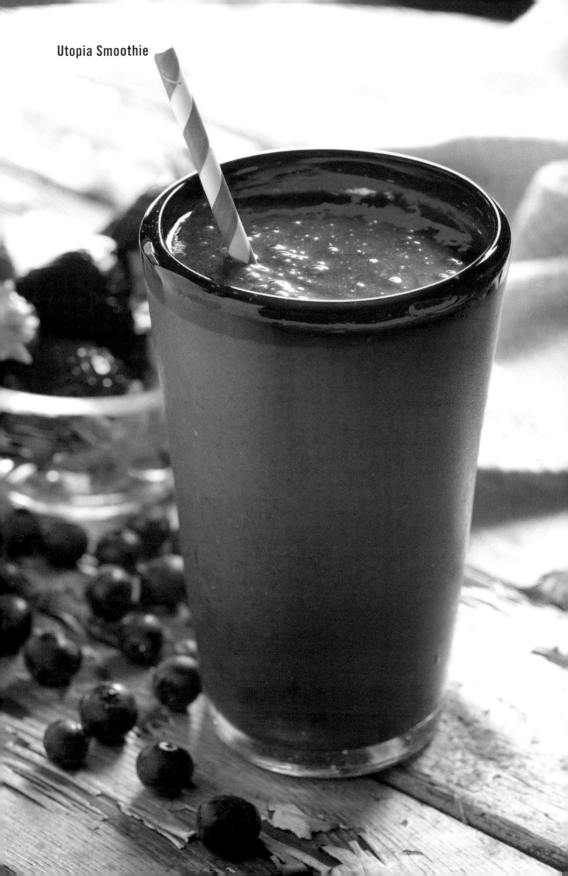

Utopia Smoothie

1

HOW THE BODY DETOXIFIES

The human body is one of the most amazing machines ever created. Complicated and resilient, at times fragile and temperamental, the body carries out tens of thousands of processes every minute of every day. One of the most important is eliminating toxic substances that accumulate in its tissues. If left undisturbed, these toxins could cause all types of harm and eventually death. The body has its own detoxification system to make sure chemicals, metabolic waste products, and dangerous free-radical molecules are adequately neutralized and removed from the body often as waste elimination.

Toxic substances are everywhere, and the vast majority of them are invisible. Sure, we see the murky fumes of pollution, whether from mining plants or car exhaust, and this is why most people tend to focus on environmental toxins. But there are many that are formed right inside of our bodies through the normal chemical reactions of daily living that can be equally dangerous. While the word *detoxification* has become quite trendy over the last decade and has taken on various meanings, simply put, detoxification refers to the process of eliminating toxins, potentially harmful substances that can lead to bad health if allowed to accumulate.

The body does a tremendous job of detoxifying on its own. It possesses four major organs that get the job done extremely well. The liver, lungs, skin, and kidneys are major cleansers; when healthy, they are programmed to do their jobs automatically. The digestive system—while not an organ but an entire system—gets a deserved honorable mention as it too is critical in eliminating toxins, whether through the process of vomiting or rectal elimination.

So if the body does such a great job of cleansing itself, why should you undertake a cleanse? There are many things beyond enhancing the body's detox systems that a cleanse can do. It can increase energy levels, promote weight loss, reduce cholesterol levels, and lower blood pressure. Beyond these physical and physiological parameters, a cleanse can also be positive from a mental standpoint. A cleanse requires discipline, focus, and honesty.

The SHRED Power Cleanse is designed to help you not just reset your nutritional and exercise routines but also clear your head and find a zone of mental sharpness and self-discovery. People who have done cleanses often speak about how much weight they've lost, but they also report how much more vigorous they feel and how they have reduced cravings for less healthy foods that might taste great but have a negative impact on their health.

Food/Beverage Detoxification

Various foods help the body in its natural detoxification process in many ways. The liver is the body's major detoxification organ, a place where the blood is cleaned and toxins are extracted and either neutralized or prepared for elimination. Various enzymes that can enhance the liver's cytochrome P450 system, which is largely responsible for the cleansing process, exist in foods.

Antioxidants are another major group of phytonutrients that are critical in helping the body fight disease and remove toxins that if left unabated could accumulate and cause injury. Antioxidants can neutralize molecules called *free radicals* that are sometimes ingested and other times simple by-products of normal processes in the body. These free radicals can be extremely harmful; if the body was not adept at eliminating them, life-threatening diseases such as cancer, atherosclerosis, asthma, diabetes, and inflammatory joint disease might develop. Antioxidants make these free radicals ineffective and help prepare them for final elimination. They too are contained in food.

Fiber is another key cleansing ingredient found in food. It's important for gastrointestinal health and easy to find in many foods, most notably in fruits, vegetables, and legumes. Fiber helps regulate bowel movements, and it can draw out all types of chemicals as it moves undigested through the gastrointestinal tract and is eventually eliminated from the body. On a daily basis, most people should consume 21 to 38 grams, depending on their age and gender. Any successful cleansing program needs to make sure it is abundant in fiber.

Water is the most important fluid that we consume and the greatest enhancer of a body cleanse. Along with air, it's the most important thing in life. At least 70 percent of our body weight is comprised of water. Water assists in the body's ability to neutralize toxins and eliminate them, whether through the skin via sweating or through the urinary tract, which includes the kidneys.

How much water do you need? The answer varies depending on the source, some saying as little as 6 cups to as much as half of your weight in water. For example, if you weigh 200 pounds, some suggest as much as 12.5 cups on a daily basis to assist in a natural cleansing process.

Exercise Detoxification

Most people don't think of exercise as a means of cleansing, but overlooking its detoxifying potential is a mistake. Exercise increases lung function, and the lungs in turn filter out toxins and other undesirable matter.

Sweating during exercise is another way that the body eliminates the undesirable toxic substances. It's all about the skin, which is our largest organ.

Exercise increases our body's circulation, which allows for better mobilization and elimination of toxic substances that might have been ingested or simply were created during our body's normal physiologic functioning. Exercise also increases the flow of lymph, a clear fluid that contains white blood cells and circulates throughout the body, helping to remove bacteria, undigested proteins from tissues, and other unwanted matter. The more you exercise, the more the lymph fluid circulates between the lymph nodes, which serve as filters to help purify the blood and lymph.

Fatty tissue located under the skin can serve as a reservoir for the storage of toxic chemicals. One of the advantages of exercise is that it can reduce this fatty tissue, thus allowing the toxins to be released. Once these toxins are no longer stored, they can be captured by the body's natural cleansing organs—the liver, kidneys, and gastrointestinal tract—and eliminated.

Sleep Detoxification

Sleep is not often thought of in detox programs, but its role can be essential and should not be ignored. Sleep is critical primarily because it allows our bodies to get restored. This just doesn't happen at a mental wellness level, but at the minute physiological level. During unconsciousness, a series of thousands of reactions repair the body, cleanse the body, and ready the body for another period of wakefulness—and all of the energy and work that it demands.

One of the primary functions of sleep is that toxins in our body are processed by various organs as energy is restored. During sleep, you are not carrying on daily functions of living such as talking, reading, walking, and eating. The body takes advantage of this time to redirect its resources to recalibrate and reset so that it's ready to handle the next stressful period of wakefulness. By stress I don't mean anxiety about a test or paying the bills or getting to work on time in rush hour traffic. Just standing up out of bed in the morning and brushing your teeth and listening to the radio creates stresses on our body's internal environment that need to be handled and addressed so that their cumulative effect doesn't restrict our ability to function.

How much sleep do we need? That's the million-dollar question. The precise number varies depending on the source, but in general it's believed to be between 6 and 8 hours for optimal health. But sleep requirement is largely idiosyncratic and can be different for everyone. Some might need more, but very few can get by effectively on less. The key is that you get enough so you're not sluggish after you get going in the morning, and you want to make sure you don't find yourself so out of energy that you need a nap in the middle of the day. The most important thing is to listen to your body. If you're not feeling restored, or your mind is cloudy and you're not carrying out tasks at the high level that you know you can, you could be sleep deprived.

2

THE SHRED POWER INGREDIENTS

One of the goals of the SHRED Power Cleanse is to consume more foods that are nutrition powerhouses. This means they're loaded with phytonutrients but have relatively few calories. Instead of getting the proverbial bang for your buck, the goal is to get the best bang for your calorie. The eleven power ingredients in this chapter—bee pollen, blueberries, chia seeds, ginger, flaxseed, hemp seed, kale, rolled oats, spinach, strawberries, and Swiss chard—have wonderful health-promoting properties strong as individuals but even greater when combined. You will eat other foods over the next fourteen days, but it's important to highlight the power ingredients because they truly are nutritional all-stars that will do everything from enhance your body's natural cleansing abilities to increase your energy and feeling of vitality.

Supplements are extremely popular for people who are trying to improve their health or augment their nutritional intake when they feel like they are deficient in certain vitamins or minerals. For many people supplements are important and they need to take them. But not everyone who takes supplements actually needs them. People who consistently eat well-balanced meals are typically getting all of the vitamins and minerals they need through their food. Clean, natural foods are the best way to load up on all of the phytonutrients that are critical for a long and healthy life. Yes, you can get some of this in a bottle, but taking it in from your plate is almost always the safest and most optimal method. The list below is not comprehensive, but an example of the types of super foods you will be consuming on the plan that will load you up on disease-fighting, energizing, satiating nutrients.

Bee Pollen

Bees collect pollen from flowers; it's the food that provides nourishment to baby bees. Claims that it is a magical ingredient for weight loss are unsubstantiated and in the past led to a cottage industry of bee supplements that promised amazing results on the scale. What science does show us, however, is that bee pollen is one of nature's most nourishing foods, with approximately 40 percent of its composition being protein, greater than any other animal source. It also contains free amino acids and vitamins, including the B-complex and folic acid. Scientists consider bee pollen to be a complete food, full of all the essential elements needed for life. Some European studies looked at whether bee pollen contained enough nutrients to sustain life. Researchers found that in fact one can live on bee pollen and water alone.

Although there are anecdotal reports that natural bee pollen can increase energy and aid in weight loss, there is little in the way of scientific evidence to support the claim, and the supplement industry is a largely unregulated industry. This is why it's important to proceed with caution when selecting the brand of bee pollen that you purchase and the source. Like anything else we consume, there are risks such as allergic reactions with the overconsumption of bee pollen, so that should be taken into consideration and consumption should be moderate. Some bee pollen supplements have been at the center of great controversy, with the FDA warning that some bee pollen products marketed for weight loss may actually threaten your health. For the purpose of the cleanse, we are not using these types of supplements, rather we're choosing organic bee pollen granules that can be added to your smoothie in small amounts. You will not taste the pollen, but it's possible that your body could experience its large nutritional potential.

Blueberries

Blueberries stand second only to strawberries as the most popular berries in the world. More species of blueberries are native to North America than to any other continent. The United States supplies over half of all blueberries to the world. Blueberries have a wonderful taste that can be sweet at times and tart at others. Their rich dark color practically screams healthy, and they are a great addition to smoothies, shakes, fruit salad, or yogurt. Blueberries are a super food because of their high nutritional value relative to their low number of calories. Just like their cousins, the strawberries, they are loaded with antioxidant phytonutrients such as anthocyanins, flavonols, and resveratrol, and with hydroxybenzoic acids.

A cup of blueberries will only cost about 84 calories, a bargain considering all of the health-promoting nutrients that it contains. Blueberries' peak availability runs from May to October, but they can be purchased all year round. Because the skin of the blueberry is consumed, you might consider purchasing organic to avoid the possibility of pesticide residue. The likelihood of encountering chemicals when consuming nonorganic blueberries, however, is relatively small because the cleaning process leaves very little if any of the pesticide as most of the chemicals are washed away. Don't be afraid to use frozen berries because they are excellent in smoothies and shakes, and they retain their nutritional benefits when frozen. While fresh provides maximal nutrition, frozen fruits and vegetables still retain the vast majority of their phytonutrients that deliver important health benefits.

Chia Seeds

Chia seeds are one of the healthiest foods on the planet. They come from the flowering plant *Salvia hispanica,* part of the mint family, and are indigenous to Mexico and parts of South America. Their seeds are tiny and can be white, dark brown, or black. Their nutritional value is enormous. One ounce of chia seeds contains 9.8 grams of fiber and 4.7 grams of protein, as well as calcium, iron, magnesium, potassium, manganese, phosphorous, omega-3 fatty acids, and omega-6 fatty acids.

The protein in chia seeds is complete, containing all nine of the essential amino acids. The Aztecs and Mayans are believed to have eaten the seeds to increase their sustainable energy. In fact, the word *chia* is the ancient Mayan word for strength. Its ability to stabilize blood sugar levels so that they don't rise too quickly can lead to the prevention of increased belly fat. The Cleveland Clinic has reported that chia seeds have also been shown to improve blood pressure in diabetics and might work to increase the levels of high-density lipoprotein (HDL), which is the healthy cholesterol, while lowering low-density lipoprotein (LDL), which is the bad cholesterol, and triglycerides.

Chia seeds can be added easily to your smoothie or shake. Because they are tasteless, they won't have any impact on the flavor of your drink or food. They can also be added to salads or toast, adding nutritional value while remaining flavor-neutral. Some people like to soak chia seeds from 15 minutes to an hour in warm water before using them because they are excellent at absorption and will increase in size. Theoretically, this larger size could mean earlier fullness as the chia seeds are believed to continue to expand and consume more volume, leaving less room for other foods.

Flaxseed

The tiny flaxseed from the *Linum usitatissimum* plant has been cultivated for thousands of years in Mediterranean and Middle Eastern countries. Now grown in other parts of the world, the seed is often dried and crushed and used to make different grades of flaxseed oil. Although tiny in size, the seed is large in nutrition. It contains a large amount of heart-healthy omega-3 fatty acids, as well as vitamin B1, copper, manganese, magnesium, phosphorous, and selenium. It also contains fiber, which adds to its prominent role in enhancing the body's natural cleansing processes.

Flaxseed is easy to add to your smoothie, but be mindful that it can result in a slightly seedy texture to the drink. Those who prefer to have a smoother texture might opt for flaxseed oil. This substitution does alter the nutritional profile; the oil still has the important omega-3 fats but no longer contains fiber. The antioxidant and antiinflammatory properties of flaxseed are largely due to its lignans, fiber-like compounds that provide its health-enhancing effects. When choosing a flaxseed oil, make sure you choose an unfiltered one so that all of the lignans and other important nutrients are preserved.

Ginger

Ginger is one of those special ingredients that pack a big punch in a small quantity. Aromatic, spicy, and pungent at the same time, ginger makes its contribution felt for almost no calories. Originating some two thousand years ago on the Asian continent, ginger is now grown all over the world. Its use in ancient times included fighting inflammation, bacterial illnesses, and flatulence. It contains several essential oils, including gingerols, which help reduce pain, lower fevers, and improve the movement of the intestines. Ginger's effect on increasing gastrointestinal movement contributes to the cleansing process because it enhances the transport of food and associated toxins through the gut so they can be removed from the body via elimination.

Although the amount of ginger used in smoothies might be small, it still contains many phytonutrients, including folate, vitamin C, potassium, calcium, magnesium, phosphorous, and manganese. A study out of Columbia University looked at the role of ginger in weight management. Researchers found that adding a ginger beverage to the diet made the subjects feel fuller after a meal and less likely to eat more later.

Fresh ginger is easy to use. Simply peel the skin and mince the ginger. One-eighth to ½ of a teaspoon is typically enough to add to your shake or smoothie and gives it a little spicy kick.

Hemp Seed

Hemp is one of the world's most nutritious plants. It is part of the genus *Cannabis* and is cultivated for its fiber and seeds. Hemp is a cannabis plant, but it's often confused with the other cannabis plants that are grown and used for the recreational drugs marijuana and hashish. The hemp plant doesn't have the mind-altering capabilities of its cousins, rather it is significant for its health-advancing abilities. The hemp seed is the edible part of the plant and is bursting with nutrition. Some scientists have gone so far as to call this seed one of the most balanced, natural sources of nonanimal complete protein, amino acids, and essential fats that can be found in nature. The protein found in hemp seeds is easily digestible and of high quality. Among a long list of its nutrients are fiber, iron, calcium, omega-3 fatty acids, omega-6 fatty acids, vitamin E, vitamin D, vitamin A, and a presence of the B vitamins.

Proteins are essential for life. The body has the ability to make some proteins but needs to get others from food. Protein is critical in building and repairing tissue and can also be used for a source of energy, just like fats and carbohydrates. Proteins are made from a collection of amino acids that are like building blocks. The body can make some of these amino acids (nonessential), while there are others (essential) that the body must get through food. Complete proteins contain all of the nine essential amino acids. Incomplete proteins lack one or more of the nine essential amino acids. Hemp seed is one of the few non-animal sources of complete protein, a small group that also includes quinoa, soybeans, and buckwheat.

Kale

Kale is on the top of all the super foods lists. Although finding new fame, it's an old plant thought to date back to 600 BCE. It's full of phytonutrients, including vitamin C, vitamin A, vitamin K, folate, quercetin (which fights inflammation and prevents plaque formation in the arteries), and sulforaphane (cancer-fighting compound). Low in calories, kale provides an appreciable amount of fiber and protein. Its deep dark-green color comes from the carotenoids lutein and zea-xanthin.

There are several types of kale, including curly, dinosaur (lacinato or Tuscan), and ornamental. Curly kale has a fibrous stalk; deep green coloring; and ruffled, curly leaves. Dinosaur kale has dark blue-green leaves with a shiny texture and has a slightly sweeter taste than curly kale. Ornamental kale has leaves that can be green, white, or purple. It tends to have a mellower flavor, but is usually used as a garnish or for food decoration as opposed to being eaten.

Rolled Oats

Oats are typically associated with the hot, thick cereal that warms your insides on a cold winter morning. It's time to expand that image: oats are one of the healthiest foods in the world and are great at every meal. An exemplary whole grain—it contains all three parts (germ, bran, and endosperm)—oats are bursting with phytonutrients that not only help with the process of cleansing but also can help stabilize blood sugars and lower cholesterol. Oats do a great job of delivering health-promoting micronutrients, including manganese, molybdenum, phosphorous, copper, biotin, vitamin B1, magnesium, chromium, and zinc. Just a quarter-cup of oats contains an astounding 5 grams of fiber and 6 grams of protein, making them a terrific addition to a smoothie or shake.

There are many varieties of oats to choose from, including whole oat groats, which are not the most popular and take the longest to cook. There are the popular steel-cut oats, which are often called Irish oatmeal. These are whole groats that have been cut into 2 or 3 pieces with a sharp blade. They cook faster because their small size allows water to penetrate more easily. The recipes in this book call for old-fashioned oats, also called rolled oats. These are formed by steaming whole oat groats and then rolling them into flakes. This allows them to stay fresh longer and helps them cook faster. Quick or instant oats are made by rolling the rolled oats even thinner and/or steaming them longer. The nutrition remains the same, but the texture changes, making them smoother and more desirable to some.

Spinach

There's a reason why the cartoon character Popeye was never too far from his strength-magnifying can of spinach. Popeye wasn't a scientist, but he must've known that the green spinach leaves are one of the most nutrient dense vegetables in nature. Vitamins A, B1, B2, B6, C, E, K, and folate, as well as important minerals such as manganese, magnesium, iron, copper, calcium, potassium, zinc, and selenium are packed into the leaves. The powerful nutritional punch that spinach delivers comes at very little calorie cost—only 41 per cup. Part of the genus *Chenopodium* (chenopods), spinach is a good source of cleansing fiber, just like its cousins Swiss chard and beets.

Spinach has a high concentration of health-enhancing phytonutrients, such as a host of flavonoids, as well as the carotenoids beta-carotene, zeaxanthin, and lutein, which give it strong antioxidant properties. Choosing the freshest leaves is important, so make sure the stems don't have any signs of yellowing and the leaves are tender and fresh-appearing rather than bruised and wilted. Add some to your smoothies or salads or simply boil them, then toss it in a bowl with a light dressing. Spinach is versatile, easy to find, and a great addition to any cleanse.

Strawberries

Sweet, fragrant, and a rush of wonderful red, the strawberry is regarded as the most popular berry fruit in the world. Once considered to be a luxury item because they were delicate, tender, and easily perishable, everyone around the world now enjoys strawberries. Strawberries are jam-packed with nutrients. Extremely high in vitamin C, they also contain manganese, iodine, folate, copper, potassium, magnesium, and omega-3 fats. With approximately 46 calories per cup, strawberries also contain 3 grams of fiber and 1 gram of protein.

Strawberries seem custom-made for helping the body rid itself of unwanted toxins. They are full of a diverse array of nutrients that function as antioxidants as well as anti-inflammatories. Anthocyanins, flavonols, tannins, resveratrol, and hydroxybenzoic acids (with their anticancer properties) are just some of the powerful health-promoting phytonutrients hidden within the sweet redness of strawberries.

Swiss Chard

This leafy green vegetable, identified in the modern era by a Swiss botanist but native to and extremely popular in the Mediterranean region, is a nutritional powerhouse. It belongs to the same family as beets and spinach but with a slightly bitter and saltier flavor. Swiss chard contains substantial amounts of vitamin K, vitamin A, vitamin C, magnesium, copper, manganese, potassium, vitamin E, iron, and fiber. It also contains at least thirteen different antioxidants, including one that can be heart-protective and another that has been shown to help regulate blood sugars.

With 1 cup of chard containing only 35 calories but donating 3 grams of fiber and 3 grams of protein to the cause, it is an excellent nutritional contributor to smoothies and shakes. Part of cleansing involves scavenging up disease-causing molecules such as free radicals. Antioxidant flavonoids such as beta-carotene, alpha-carotene, lutein, and zeaxanthin, which are found in chard, are helpful in neutralizing these free-radical toxins, thus rendering them harmless.

3

HOW THE SHRED POWER CLEANSE WORKS

The SHRED Power Cleanse is unique because it doesn't obligate you to exclusively consume drinks. You can also eat salads, soups, and snacks. Each day of this two-week plan is clearly laid out for you so that you know what you need to consume and how you need to consume it. Another unique aspect of the cleanse is that it includes exercise. Just eating well is only part of what you can do to enhance your body's natural cleansing mechanisms. Exercising is another way that the body is able to eliminate toxic substances, so this part of the program should be treated with the same regard as the meals and snacks.

The plan is two weeks long. The margin for error is not as large as it would be if you were on a twenty-one day or longer cleanse. Yet, while there's not a lot of room for error, the program is designed so that it's not highly restrictive or penalizing. Just like my other SHRED programs (SHRED Diet and Super SHRED) this cleanse has been engineered with three major principles in mind. It's accessible—the foods and ingredients called for are not rare or so unique that it's diffi-

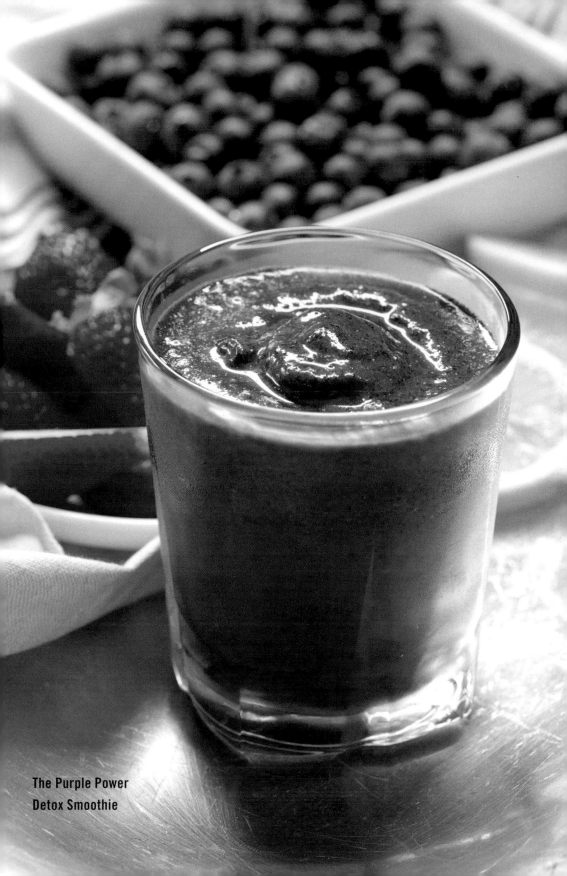

The Purple Power
Detox Smoothie

cult to locate them or incorporate them into your program. It's realistic. Who wants to spend two weeks drinking weird-tasting beverages? The smoothies and shakes on this program are tasty and full of a broad range of flavors. They carry a sufficient amount of calories to keep you satisfied, and they are extremely easy to make right in your own kitchen. And it's flexible—it can fit well into other types of programs that you might be following. Whether you are a vegetarian, a vegan, following a paleo lifestyle (based on foods our human ancestors might likely have eaten—meat, fish, nuts, seeds, fruits, and vegetables), or following a "right-carb" program (eating healthy carbohydrates), you can still do the cleanse effectively and not disrupt your overall plan. Remember, this cleanse is only two weeks long and not indefinite, so it should be viewed more as an addition or transition to a healthier way of eating.

There are all kinds of ingredients that can go into making a smoothie, and in many cases our preferences for taste and texture can make a difference in whether we choose one over another. But when it comes to a total package that includes taste, texture, and nutritional power, there's nothing like the Purple Smoothie. Easy to make, a natural energy booster, and with ingredients that are available all year round, these smoothies can pack in half of your day's recommended servings of fruits and vegetables in just 1 glass.

These Purple Smoothies are sweet, creamy, and full of phytonutrients that include a healthy dose of fiber and protein. Blueberries form the nutrient backbone of this smoothie, but a Purple Smoothie also packs in kale, spinach, or other leafy greens whose presence you would never guess at because of the deep rich-purple color and the sweet taste. These drinks are jam-packed with disease-fighting and health-promoting antioxidants that work overtime in your body to keep you out of harm's way. Satisfying on many levels and full of natural ingredients, the Purple Smoothie will leave you feeling full and vigorous.

Nutrition Guidelines

Each day of the program is written in a specific order that you are to follow. Be mindful of that particular day, and don't assume that it's the same as the other days. Some days are similar to each other, while others can be quite different. Each day will have two or more liquid meal replacements in the form of a smoothie, shake, or soup. Try your best to make your own smoothies and shakes with the recipes provided in chapter 7. All of the recipes make two servings, so simply consume one for that particular meal slot and take the other serving with you to drink later or store it in your fridge. Smoothies can be frozen and consumed later at your convenience.

You might not always be in a situation where you can make your own smoothie or shake, so you will need to get them from a retailer. It's simply not possible for me to review every brand of smoothie or shake that exists, but there are simple guidelines you should follow when deciding what to buy. Any smoothie you purchase from a third party must be 300 calories or less and contain no added sugars. If you like smoothies on the sweeter side, ask for ½ teaspoon of raw organic honey to be added.

If you need to purchase a premade shake, please be mindful that protein shakes have lots of calories. Your store-bought shake also needs to be 300 calories or less, and contain natural ingredients and no added sugars or artificial sweeteners. Adding a tablespoon or less of organic protein powder is completely fine, but choose one that is genuinely natural, which means that it is of high quality and contains no artificial ingredients such as artificial sweeteners, preservatives, and other unnatural or known harmful chemicals.

Salads are an important part of the SHRED Power Cleanse. They are a great way to get your mouth chewing again—a simple pleasure in life that's easy to take for granted until you've only been drinking your meals for a few days. Other cleanses don't allow salads, but the

SHRED Power Cleanse integrates them into your daily regimen because salads can be a great nutritional source and enhance your body's cleanse. The key, however, is to make sure your salads are CLEAN! This means only raw ingredients and dressing that is low in fat and calories. You'll find 2 simple dressing recipes that you can make in 5 minutes in the Appendix. They are tasty and free of the synthetic chemicals that we are aiming to avoid during these two weeks. Your salad should primarily contain leafy greens, tomatoes, olives, cucumbers, onions, and peppers. Your salad can contain as many or as few of these ingredients as you like. You can also add 2 tablespoons of organic or natural shredded cheese—which can deliver a little calcium and protein to your salad—or sprinkle on 8 to 10 nuts.

If you find yourself in a situation where the day's guidelines call for a smoothie, but all you can get is a shake, go ahead and make the switch. If a particular day has a smoothie, clean salad, and shake in the plan, but at the time you're supposed to be eating a shake and you can only access a salad, feel free to make the switch. The bottom line: follow the plan as closely as possible, but life happens and sometimes you need the flexibility to make swaps. The program will accommodate this.

Snacks are important in all SHRED programs, especially in the Power Cleanse. The snacks listed during the daily plans have been specially selected. You are heavily discouraged from making substitutions in this part of the program. Eating clean and reaping the results relies on making smart choices. Snacks can be an extremely tricky part of one's diet, especially since there are so many ingredients that manufacturers include and don't disclose—or perhaps do disclose, but the names of the ingredients are too complicated to understand. Snacks are another opportunity for you to chew again, but they are not supposed to be an opportunity to load up on calories and synthetic ingredients. If you miss a snack, do not double up during the next snack slot. It's missed and you move on to the next item.

Exercise

Each day has a recommended amount of exercise that you are to complete for the day. While foods are an excellent way to enhance your body's natural cleansing processes, they are not working alone. Exercising is important to maximize your results. Not only will it enhance weight loss, improve circulation, and increase sweating elimination of toxins, it will keep your body and mind primed for peak performance. When the plan calls for a certain amount of exercise for that day, it also gives you flexibility in how you complete your exercise. Maybe you have not been exercising on a regular basis and now the program is recommending that you do some. Rather than doing the entire exercise session at once, you should consider breaking it up into two sessions. So if you have a 30-minute session for the day, you can break it up into two different 15-minute sessions. Remember, the key is not just the amount of exercise you do, but the intensity of the exercise. It's important to get your heart rate up and perform at a moderate level of intensity.

The exercise recommended during these two weeks revolves around cardiovascular exercises. This, however, doesn't mean you can't do some resistance training. If you want to add this to the day's listed exercise recommendation, feel free to do so, but don't *replace* the cardio exercises with resistance training. Adding two or three 30-minute resistance training sessions to your week's workout schedule is completely fine, and this can help increase your metabolism, increase your lean muscle, and sculpt your body.

High-intensity interval training (HIIT) is excellent for burning calories in a short period of time. This type of exercising is also called *burst training*; there's a short period of high exertion followed by a rest period, then back to the high exertion and another rest period. For example, imagine sprinting as hard as you can for 30 seconds and then walking for 20 seconds, then going back to sprinting for 30 seconds.

This switching between high-exertion intervals and low-exertion intervals drives your metabolism through the roof, and unlike more traditional exercising—such as jogging on a treadmill at a steady pace for 20 minute—you can actually burn calories at a higher rate up to 24 hours after the exercise is complete.

There are many HIIT workouts that are effective, and you should try what interests you. I have developed two workouts—the SHRED 27 Burn and the SHRED 15 Burn. The SHRED 27 Burn is a 27-minute workout that doesn't require any machinery. All you need is a small amount of floor space and a bottle of water. The SHRED 15 Burn is a 15-minute workout that uses 3 pieces of fitness equipment almost all well-equipped gyms will possess—stationary bike, elliptical, and treadmill. If you would like to try these workouts, simply go to www.shredlife.com and look in the SHRED store.

Meal Schedule

So much attention is paid to what we eat and the quantity we consume. Keeping watch on calorie intake is an important component to eating healthy and making wise decisions. But calories only tell part of the story. When you eat can make a big difference also. Science has shown that it's more advantageous to distribute calories as evenly as possible throughout the day. This even distribution prevents a sharp spike of hormones such as insulin, which can lead to a rapid movement of sugar and other nutrients into the cells and potentially lead to weight gain.

Each week of the SHRED Power Cleanse has a meal schedule guide that you should follow. The goal is to prevent you from overindulging during meals and being hungry between meals. Your schedule should be based on when you wake up and when you go to sleep. Sometimes you might need to adjust your eating times based on your day's activities, but try your best to keep as close to the schedule as possible. Your body appreciates regularity when it comes to nourishment, and your mood can often be tied to your body feeling undernourished or over-nourished.

After the Cleanse

You've completed the cleanse: What's next? Some individuals might be inspired to continue the cleanse for another two-week cycle. If you are up to the task physically and mentally, go ahead and do so. Some of you have now learned the positive impact clean eating can have on your weight as well as your energy level. If you would like to keep this going and adopt a healthier eating lifestyle and lose weight, then you should try my previous book, *SHRED: The Revolutionary Diet*. For those who want to continue to eat and move healthier, but would like to lose weight at a faster clip, you should try *Super SHRED: The Big Results Diet*. Both programs incorporate some of the principles of the SHRED Power Cleanse.

Now that you have done the entire cleanse and plan on adopting healthier eating habits, you might want to do a tune-up period-ically. It would be akin to taking your car to the mechanic to make sure the brakes are in good order, fluid levels are balanced, and the oil changed. Chapter 6 contains your tune-up: the SHRED Power Weekend Cleanse. This three-day plan is just enough to rejuvenate you after a tough week of unhealthy eating and drinking or when you find yourself getting sluggish or your weight creeping up.

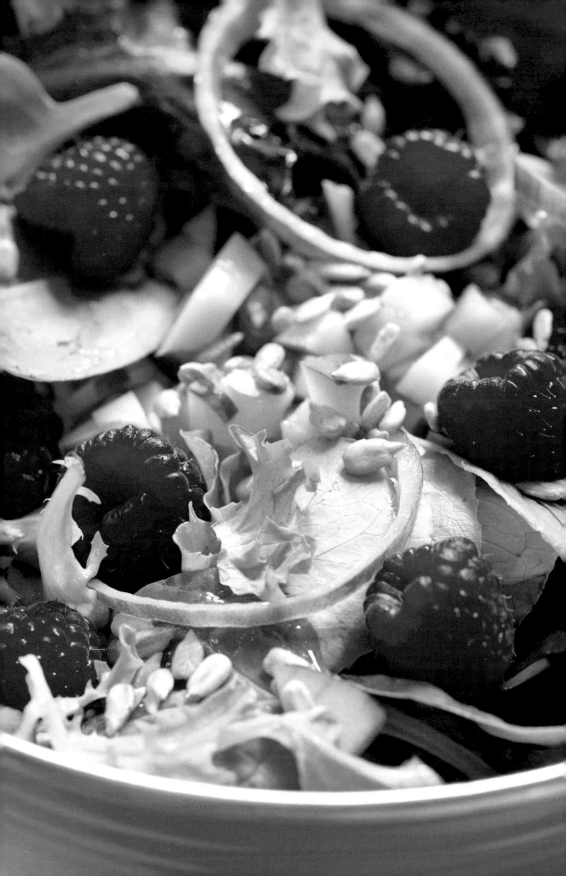

4

WEEK 1: LAUNCH

The SHRED Power Cleanse doesn't take its time to get you in orbit. Right from the beginning, you will start to cleanse your system of all types of toxins that have been accumulating in your body. Because this is only a two-week program, you really have to commit yourself. There is little room to deviate from the program because your body needs to avoid unhealthy foods that might taste good going down but can do a lot of damage once inside. If you have an allergy to something described on the menu, by all means make a smart substitution. For example, if you're allergic to cow's milk, then try soy or goat's milk.

The timing of meals during the cleanse is extremely important. Make sure you don't skip, and try to hit your time slots as accurately as possible so that your body is properly refueled and you don't start feeling deprived. If for some reason—such as being on a plane—you miss your meal or snack time, move on to the next meal or snack at the normal time. Don't double up a meal or snack, and don't disrupt the remainder of the schedule because you missed a slot earlier.

Exercise is an important component of your detoxification. Do as much of what is suggested as you can. If you don't hit all of the exercise bench marks, that doesn't mean you won't successfully cleanse. You'll cleanse faster if you exercise. Exercise is definitely a cleansing accelerant: it increases blood flow; accelerates respiration so our lungs exchange bad gases for good gases; and leads to sweating, which is another way the body cleanses. Exercise is important for a complete program so that your cleansing is maximized.

Power Snack

Each day you are allowed an extra snack. This snack is meant to power you through the times when you really are hungry or feel the need for a jolt of energy. This snack is meant to be used ONLY if you need it. Don't just eat it because you want an extra snack. This Power Snack is available to you on any day of the program, at any time, but you're only allowed a maximum of one per day. Be smart with your Power Snack, save it for a stretch between meals or at a time between a snack and meal when you are really hungry. Try not to eat it at the same time as a designated snack or a time that's really close to your last snack. For your power snack, you must choose from the following list:

10 baby carrots (2 tablespoons of low-calorie dressing
   or natural hummus optional)
1 cup of cherries
10 cherry tomatoes
1 boiled egg with seasoning (sprinkle of salt allowed)
1 piece of fruit
1 cup of any type of berries
1 cup of any type of melon chunks
1 cup of plain air-popped popcorn
1½ cups of sugar snap peas
½ cup of shelled edamame beans

3 tablespoons sunflower seeds in their shells

20 almonds

1 small banana (optional: 1 tablespoon organic or natural peanut butter)

1 celery stalk (optional: 1 tablespoon organic or natural peanut butter)

Eating Schedule

Space your meals throughout the day. Eat your first meal within an hour of getting up and your last meal no closer than 90 minutes before going to bed. Below is a sample meal schedule for someone who wakes up at 7 A.M. Your meal schedule will look different based on the time you wake up. Try your best to hit the time as closely as you can, but if you don't, you have a 45-minute grace period. Avoid skipping meals, but if you are 45 minutes past the time you were supposed to eat a meal or snack, then move on and make sure you don't double up on the next snack or meal to compensate. If in the later part of the day you find yourself getting hungry, eat a piece of fruit.

Awake	Morning Smoothie	Snack 1	Shake	Clean Salad	Evening Smoothie	Snack 2
7 A.M.	8 A.M.	9:30 A.M.	12:00 P.M.	3:00 P.M.	6:30 P.M.	8:30 P.M.

*Don't forget your Power Snack is available to you at any time.

GUIDELINE REMINDERS

▶ All shakes and smoothies are 12 ounces (a cup and a half).

▶ All salads are fruits and veggies; only 3 tablespoons fat-free or low-fat, low-calorie clean dressing.

- Feel free to add 1 tablespoon of organic protein powder to each shake (organic hemp or whey).
- If you need to make substitutions, make smart ones that don't increase calorie counts.
- Make sure 1 of your smoothies is the SHRED Purple Power Detox Smoothie.
- Make sure all nuts are unsalted.
- Where the recipe calls for a specific variety of kale, you can change to a different type of your preference.
- When recipes call for frozen berries, you can substitute with fresh berries, but be mindful that if you don't have ice or chilled liquid in the drink, it will be warm and needs to be refrigerated unless you don't mind room-temperature smoothies.
- Consume at least 6 cups of water each day. This should be plain flat or fizzy water, not flavored water with additives.
- You can replace the morning smoothie with a cup of whole grain cereal such as oatmeal. You can use ½ cup of low-fat, fat-free, skim, almond, soy, or coconut milk. One-half teaspoon of raw organic honey is allowed. You can only make this replacement three times during the week.
- You can replace a smoothie, shake, or salad with a soup 3 times during the week, but not in the same day. So you can have just one switch a day for three days of your choice on the program. You can cook your own soup or purchase one. Be careful of the ingredients so that you can keep eating as cleanly as possible. Avoid cream soups and choose broth- or tomato-based soups. If you buy canned soup, go for those marked low-sodium, and make sure they contain 480 milligrams of sodium or less. The lower the sodium count the better. Acceptable soups include but are not limited to black bean, vegetable, corn, tomato, pea, butternut squash, sweet potato, lentil, chickpea, and vegetarian (without the noodles). These soups should also be 200 calories or less.

SHRED THOUGHT: *Regardless of how great the architectural wonder, it all started with one brick or stone.* Today is only one brick. Imagine standing in front of a five-story brick building and looking at its solidity. Think about standing in front of the great Mayan Kukulkan Pyramid in the middle of Chichen Itza, Mexico, and looking at the amazing architectural feat that was accomplished between 800 CE and 900 CE without any machinery or modern construction know-how. The pyramid was built by hand one stone at a time to the height of 98 feet. That's what it's like to rebuild yourself and adopt healthy lifestyle behaviors. It starts with one day, and then comes the second and the third, and before you know it—by stringing several together—you go into weeks and months. But don't think about what the entire expanse will look like yet. Just think about this first day, which is the first brick in your beautiful new you.

TODAY'S SHRED POWER CLEANSE

Morning Smoothie

Choose a smoothie from chapter 7 to make yourself. If you're unable to make the smoothie and must purchase it, make sure the smoothie is fresh (meaning it is made by the retailer with fresh ingredients) and

not pre-packaged, contains 300 calories or less, and doesn't contain added sugar. One-half teaspoon of raw organic honey is allowed if you really need it to sweeten the taste.

You can also have a "deconstructed" smoothie. Instead of blending the ingredients, you can mix them all in a bowl and eat them. You don't need to include the liquid portion of the smoothie, but feel free to have as much of the other ingredients as you like. Don't worry, you still get the benefits of the ingredients even if they're not blended.

Snack 1

Choose one of the following:

15 baby carrot sticks
1 celery stalk cut into slices
15 cucumber slices
20 almonds
10 cherry tomatoes
Any piece of fruit
1 cup of any type of berries

Shake

In a perfect world, you will make your own shake using one of the recipes from chapter 7. I created these recipes with the program's cleansing goals in sharp focus. However, if you need to purchase a shake, make sure it is 300 calories or less, contains natural ingredients, and doesn't contain added sugars or other artificial sweeteners or synthetic chemicals. You can add protein powder to your shake, but be mindful that protein powders can add a lot of calories.

Clean Salad or Roasted Vegetables

Your salad should be made of 3 cups or less of leafy greens. You can include all or none of the following: 1 small tomato cut into slices (or

6 cherry tomatoes); 3 olives (any variety); 8 slices of cucumbers or the diced equivalent; 3 slices of onion; ¼ cup of diced red, green, or yellow pepper; ½ cup of shredded carrot. You're allowed to have 2 tablespoons of fat-free or low-fat dressing. Make sure the dressing you choose is 70 calories or less per 2 tablespoons, with a sodium content of 400 milligrams or less per 2 tablespoons. You can also make your own salad dressing very easily. Check out the simple recipes in the Appendix.

Instead of a salad, you can choose to have 2 cups or less of roasted vegetables. Your vegetables can include peppers, onions, Brussels sprouts, carrots, tomatoes, squash, zucchini, potatoes (sweet or white), beets, broccoli, mushrooms, and kale or other leafy greens. For cooking and seasoning you can use a tablespoon of olive oil, and salt and pepper and other herbs, to taste.

Evening Smoothie

Choose a smoothie from chapter 7 to make yourself. If you're unable to make the smoothie and must purchase it, make sure the smoothie is fresh (meaning it is made by the retailer with fresh ingredients) and not pre-packaged, contains 300 calories or less, and doesn't contain added sugar. One-half teaspoon of raw organic honey is allowed if you really need it to sweeten the taste.

You can also have a "deconstructed" smoothie. Instead of blending the ingredients, you can mix them all in a bowl and eat them. You don't need to include the liquid portion of the smoothie, but feel free to have as much of the other ingredients as you like. Don't worry, you still get the benefits of the ingredients even if they're not blended.

Choose one of the following for your snack. You can always have 2 tablespoons of a low-calorie balsamic vinaigrette or 3 tablespoons of a low-calorie natural hummus to dip your snack in for flavor.

15 baby carrot sticks
1 celery stalk cut into slices
15 cucumber slices
20 almonds
10 cherry tomatoes
Any piece of fruit
1 cup of any type of berries

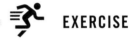 **EXERCISE**

Minimum: 30 minutes. If you want to do a little more, all the better.

You get as much out of exercise as you put into it. Exercise is not a time to socialize and simply occupy time. It's your appointment with your body to focus on improving the way it moves, feels, and looks. One of your goals in exercising should be to push yourself to work as hard as possible in a short period of time. Remember, the time listed below is not how long you are expected to be present in an exercise environment such as the gym; rather, it is meant to be how much time you are actually exercising. The clock doesn't start until you begin moving and it stops when you stop. While a gym can be convenient for many, you don't have to go to a gym to exercise. You can do it right in your own backyard, in your bedroom, basement, or wherever you have floor space. Try to vary your workouts: choose one that's different from the last one you did. Below you will find some 15-minute interval exercises to try. For example, if the program calls for 30 minutes, you can do 15 minutes of fast walking/jogging on the treadmill and 15 minutes riding the stationary or a mobile bike. You can also do 30 minutes of riding the stationary or mobile bike. But remember, regardless of what you choose, the intensity of your exercise is important. It's your decision how to break up the exercise, but understand that changing your routine is typically more advantageous than simply doing the same type of exercise for the entire workout.

You can do either the SHRED 27 Burn workout or the SHRED 15 Burn workout or choose a combination of the items below to fulfill your exercise requirement of 30 minutes. Check out the SHRED workout videos at www. shredlife.com.

15 minutes walking/running on treadmill

15 minutes on elliptical machine

15 minutes walking/jogging outside

15 minutes swimming laps

15 minutes on stationary or mobile bicycle

15 minutes on rowing machine

15 minutes of spinning class

15 minutes of Zumba

15 minutes on stair climber

15 minutes of treadmill intervals (fast walk/jog alternating with slow walk/slow jog)

225 jump rope revolutions

15 minutes of any other high-intensity cardio

JOURNAL ENTRY WEEK 1, DAY 1

What Went Well?

_____

_____

_____

What Didn't Go Well?

_____

_____

_____

What Did You Feel Throughout the Day Emotionally and Physically?

_____

_____

_____

Goals You Met Today

_____

_____

_____

Today's Inspiration

_____

_____

_____

SHRED THOUGHT: *Even with the best of skills, the difference between succeeding and failing comes down to attitude.* Studies have clearly shown that people who are optimistic are happier and live longer. Studies also show that they tend to reach their goals with greater frequency. How you mentally approach the tasks before you today and over these next two weeks will greatly determine your success with the SHRED Power Cleanse. Instead of looking at something as "difficult," consider it to be "challenging." Instead of thinking about how much more exercise you have to do, think about how much exercise you've already done. A positive can-do attitude will make your tasks easier and your days faster. Rather than just getting through the day, your goal should be enjoying the day while becoming a better you.

TODAY'S SHRED POWER CLEANSE

Morning Smoothie

Choose a smoothie from chapter 7 to make yourself. If you're unable to make the smoothie and must purchase it, make sure the smoothie is fresh (meaning it is made by the retailer with fresh ingredients) and

not pre-packaged, contains 300 calories or less, and doesn't contain added sugar. One-half teaspoon of raw organic honey is allowed if you really need it to sweeten the taste.

You can also have a "deconstructed" smoothie. Instead of blending the ingredients, you can mix them all in a bowl and eat them. You don't need to include the liquid portion of the smoothie, but feel free to have as much of the other ingredients as you like. Don't worry, you still get the benefits of the ingredients even if they're not blended.

Snack 1

Make sure you drink 1 cup of plain water with your snack. The water can be flat or fizzy, but no artificial flavoring. You can squeeze a piece of citrus fruit into your water or you can drink fresh-fruit infused water by immersing sliced fruit in the water to add flavor. Try sliced strawberries, oranges, pineapple, etc.

Choose one of the following for your snack:

15 baby carrot sticks
1 celery stalk cut into slices
15 cucumber slices
20 almonds
10 cherry tomatoes
Any piece of fruit
1 cup of any type of berries

Shake

In a perfect world, you will make your own shake using one of the recipes from chapter 7. I created these recipes with the program's cleansing goals in sharp focus. However, if you need to purchase a shake, make sure it is 300 calories or less, contains natural ingredients, and doesn't contain added sugars or other artificial sweeteners or synthetic chemicals. You can add protein powder to your shake, but be mindful that protein powders can add a lot of calories.

Clean Salad

Your salad should be made of 3 cups or less of leafy greens. You can include all or none of the following: 1 small tomato cut into slices (or 6 cherry tomatoes); 3 olives (any variety); 8 slices of cucumbers or the diced equivalent; 3 slices of onion; ¼ cup of diced red, green, or yellow pepper; ½ cup of shredded carrot. You're allowed to have 2 tablespoons of fat-free or low-fat dressing. Make sure the dressing you choose is 70 calories or less per 2 tablespoons, with a sodium content of 400 milligrams or less per 2 tablespoons. You can also make your own salad dressing very easily. Check out the simple recipes in the Appendix.

Evening Smoothie

Choose a smoothie from chapter 7 to make yourself. If you're unable to make the smoothie and must purchase it, make sure the smoothie is fresh (meaning it is made by the retailer with fresh ingredients) and not pre-packaged, contains 300 calories or less, and doesn't contain added sugar. One-half teaspoon of raw organic honey is allowed if you really need it to sweeten the taste.

You can also have a "deconstructed" smoothie. Instead of blending the ingredients, you can mix them all in a bowl and eat them. You don't need to include the liquid portion of the smoothie, but feel free to have as much of the other ingredients as you like. Don't worry, you still get the benefits of the ingredients even if they're not blended.

Choose one of the following for your snack. You can always have 2 tablespoons of a low-calorie balsamic vinaigrette or 3 tablespoons of a low-calorie natural hummus to dip your snack in for flavor.

15 baby carrot sticks
1 celery stalk cut into slices
15 cucumber slices
20 almonds
10 cherry tomatoes
Any piece of fruit
1 cup of any type of berries

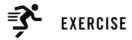 **EXERCISE**

Minimum: 45 minutes. If you want to do a little more, all the better.

You can do either the SHRED 27 Burn workout or the SHRED 15 Burn workout or choose a combination of the items below to fulfill your exercise requirement of 45 minutes. Check out the SHRED workout videos at www. shredlife.com.

15 minutes walking/running on treadmill
15 minutes on elliptical machine
15 minutes walking/jogging outside
15 minutes swimming laps
15 minutes on stationary or mobile bicycle
15 minutes on rowing machine
15 minutes of spinning class
15 minutes of Zumba
15 minutes on stair climber

15 minutes of treadmill intervals (fast walk/jog alternating with
slow walk/slow jog)

225 jump rope revolutions

15 minutes of any other high-intensity cardio

JOURNAL ENTRY WEEK 1, DAY 2

What Went Well?

_____

_____

_____

What Didn't Go Well?

_____

_____

_____

What Did You Feel Throughout the Day Emotionally and Physically?

_____

_____

_____

Goals You Met Today

_____

_____

_____

Today's Inspiration

_____

_____

_____

SHRED THOUGHT: *The second you get those stirrings that it's easier to quit, simply ask yourself why you started.* Thoughts of quitting are a completely natural response to stress, doubt, difficulty, and uncertainty. All of us have feelings of giving up at one time or another. But when you think of quitting is when you have to roll up your sleeves and fight even harder. Go back to the foundation and remind yourself of why you decided to embark on this mission. There is a constant struggle between what you know you should do and what you can do that might be easier. Remember what got you to this point and spark your determination not to turn back.

TODAY'S SHRED POWER CLEANSE

Morning Smoothie

Choose a smoothie from chapter 7 to make yourself. If you're unable to make the smoothie and must purchase it, make sure the smoothie is fresh (meaning it is made by the retailer with fresh ingredients) and not pre-packaged, contains 300 calories or less, and doesn't contain added sugar. One-half teaspoon of raw organic honey is allowed if you really need it to sweeten the taste.

You can also have a "deconstructed" smoothie. Instead of blend-

ing the ingredients, you can mix them all in a bowl and eat them. You don't need to include the liquid portion of the smoothie, but feel free to have as much of the other ingredients as you like. Don't worry, you still get the benefits of the ingredients even if they're not blended.

Snack 1

Choose one of the following for your snack:

15 baby carrot sticks
1 celery stalk cut into slices
15 cucumber slices
20 almonds
10 cherry tomatoes
Any piece of fruit
1 cup of any type of berries

Shake

In a perfect world, you will make your own shake using one of the recipes from chapter 7. I created these recipes with the program's cleansing goals in sharp focus. However, if you need to purchase a shake, make sure it is 300 calories or less, contains natural ingredients, and doesn't contain added sugars or other artificial sweeteners or synthetic chemicals. You can add protein powder to your shake, but be mindful that protein powders can add a lot of calories.

Clean Salad or Roasted Vegetables

Your salad should be made of 3 cups or less of leafy greens. You can include all or none of the following: 1 small tomato cut into slices (or 6 cherry tomatoes); 3 olives (any variety); 8 slices of cucumbers or the diced equivalent; 3 slices of onion; ¼ cup of diced red, green, or yellow pepper; ½ cup of shredded carrot. You're allowed to have 2 tablespoons of fat-free or low-fat dressing. Make sure the dressing you choose is 70 calories or less per 2 tablespoons, with a sodium content of 400 milligrams or less per 2 tablespoons. You can also make your own salad dressing very easily. Check out the simple recipes in the Appendix.

Instead of a salad, you can choose to have 2 cups or less of roasted vegetables. Your vegetables can include peppers, onions, Brussels sprouts, carrots, tomatoes, squash, zucchini, potatoes (sweet or white), beets, broccoli, mushrooms, and kale or other leafy greens. For cooking and seasoning you can use a tablespoon of olive oil, and salt and pepper and other herbs, to taste.

Evening Smoothie

Choose a smoothie from chapter 7 to make yourself. If you're unable to make the smoothie and must purchase it, make sure the smoothie is fresh (meaning it is made by the retailer with fresh ingredients) and not pre-packaged, contains 300 calories or less, and doesn't contain added sugar. One-half teaspoon of raw organic honey is allowed if you really need it to sweeten the taste.

You can also have a "deconstructed" smoothie. Instead of blending the ingredients, you can mix them all in a bowl and eat them. You don't need to include the liquid portion of the smoothie, but feel free to have as much of the other ingredients as you like. Don't worry, you still get the benefits of the ingredients even if they're not blended.

Snack 2

Choose one of the following for your snack. You can always have 2 tablespoons of a low-calorie balsamic vinaigrette or 3 tablespoons of a low-calorie natural hummus to dip your snack in for flavor.

15 baby carrot sticks
1 celery stalk cut into slices
15 cucumber slices

20 almonds

10 cherry tomatoes

Any piece of fruit

1 cup of any type of berries

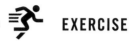 **EXERCISE**

Rest Day: Your body needs to recover in order to improve. Take this day to allow restoration.

JOURNAL ENTRY WEEK 1, DAY 3

What Went Well?

_____

_____

_____

What Didn't Go Well?

_____

_____

_____

What Did You Feel Throughout the Day Emotionally and Physically?

_____

_____

_____

Goals You Met Today

_____

_____

_____

Today's Inspiration

_____

_____

_____

SHRED THOUGHT: *No measurement exists to accurately quantify the power of the mind.* Our ability to overcome difficulties, absorb loss, continue to hope in the face of despair, and scale seemingly insurmountable obstacles depends on our mental strength and our ability to power ourselves to victory. There are legendary stories about people who have overcome days in the freezing wilderness without shelter, long periods of time drifting at sea without food, or those living in small villages walking miles to get fresh water for their family. All of these situations required physical strength, but above that mental toughness was what saved the day. You can do what you put your mind to, regardless of how tough it might be. Exercise your mental muscles.

TODAY'S SHRED POWER CLEANSE

Morning Smoothie

Choose a smoothie from chapter 7 to make yourself. If you're unable to make the smoothie and must purchase it, make sure the smoothie is fresh (meaning it is made by the retailer with fresh ingredients) and not pre-packaged, contains 300 calories or less, and doesn't contain added sugar. One-half teaspoon of raw organic honey is allowed if you really need it to sweeten the taste.

You can also have a "deconstructed" smoothie. Instead of blending the ingredients, you can mix them all in a bowl and eat them. You don't need to include the liquid portion of the smoothie, but feel free to have as much of the other ingredients as you like. Don't worry, you still get the benefits of the ingredients even if they're not blended.

Snack 1

Choose one of the following for your snack:

15 baby carrot sticks
1 celery stalk cut into slices
15 cucumber slices
20 almonds
10 cherry tomatoes
Any piece of fruit
1 cup of any type of berries

Shake

In a perfect world, you will make your own shake using one of the recipes from chapter 7. I created these recipes with the program's cleansing goals in sharp focus. However, if you need to purchase a shake, make sure it is 300 calories or less, contains natural ingredients, and doesn't contain added sugars or other artificial sweeteners or synthetic chemicals. You can add protein powder to your shake, but be mindful that protein powders can add a lot of calories.

Clean Salad

Your salad should be made of 3 cups or less of leafy greens. You can include all or none of the following: 1 small tomato cut into slices (or 6 cherry tomatoes); 3 olives (any variety); 8 slices of cucumbers or the diced equivalent; 3 slices of onion; ¼ cup of diced red, green, or yellow pepper; ½ cup of shredded carrot. You're allowed to have

2 tablespoons of fat-free or low-fat dressing. Make sure the dressing you choose is 70 calories or less per 2 tablespoons, with a sodium content of 400 milligrams or less per 2 tablespoons. You can also make your own salad dressing very easily. Check out the simple recipes in the Appendix.

Evening Smoothie

Choose a smoothie from chapter 7 to make yourself. If you're unable to make the smoothie and must purchase it, make sure the smoothie is fresh (meaning it is made by the retailer with fresh ingredients) and not pre-packaged, contains 300 calories or less, and doesn't contain added sugar. One-half teaspoon of raw organic honey is allowed if you really need it to sweeten the taste.

You can also have a "deconstructed" smoothie. Instead of blending the ingredients, you can mix them all in a bowl and eat them. You don't need to include the liquid portion of the smoothie, but feel free to have as much of the other ingredients as you like. Don't worry, you still get the benefits of the ingredients even if they're not blended.

Snack 2

Choose one of the following for your snack. You can always have 2 tablespoons of a low-calorie balsamic vinaigrette or 3 tablespoons of a low-calorie natural hummus to dip your snack in for flavor.

15 baby carrot sticks
1 celery stalk cut into slices
15 cucumber slices
20 almonds
10 cherry tomatoes
Any piece of fruit
1 cup of any type of berries

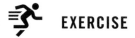

Minimum: 45 minutes. If you want to do a little more, all the better.

You can do either the SHRED 27 Burn workout or the SHRED 15 Burn workout or choose a combination of the items below to fulfill your exercise requirement of 45 minutes. Check out the SHRED workout videos at www. shredlife.com.

15 minutes walking/running on treadmill

15 minutes on elliptical machine

15 minutes walking/jogging outside

15 minutes swimming laps

15 minutes on stationary or mobile bicycle

15 minutes on rowing machine

15 minutes of spinning class

15 minutes of Zumba

15 minutes on stair climber

15 minutes of treadmill intervals (fast walk/jog alternating with slow walk/slow jog)

225 jump rope revolutions

15 minutes of any other high-intensity cardio

JOURNAL ENTRY WEEK 1, DAY 4

What Went Well?

_____

_____

_____

What Didn't Go Well?

_____

_____

_____

What Did You Feel Throughout the Day Emotionally and Physically?

_____

_____

_____

Goals You Met Today

_____

_____

_____

Today's Inspiration

_____

_____

_____

SHRED THOUGHT: *Your body is more than just something you evaluate in a mirror, it's the most beautiful and complicated machine ever created.* How you take care of this creation will determine how well it works, how much it can achieve, and how long it lasts. Like other machines with many parts that must work in unison, the body needs to be tuned up, oiled when it creaks, and cleaned on a regular basis. What you put into your body has a tremendous impact on how efficiently it works and how well it stands up to the many stresses it encounters on a daily basis. Foods and beverages that focus on natural ingredients and avoid the additives, preservatives, and other synthetic chemicals used to process foods are the best fuel to optimize health and provide the nourishment for the body's best operation.

TODAY'S SHRED POWER CLEANSE

Morning Smoothie

Choose a smoothie from chapter 7 to make yourself. If you're unable to make the smoothie and must purchase it, make sure the smoothie is fresh (meaning it is made by the retailer with fresh ingredients) and not pre-packaged, contains 300 calories or less, and doesn't contain

added sugar. One-half teaspoon of raw organic honey is allowed if you really need it to sweeten the taste.

You can also have a "deconstructed" smoothie. Instead of blending the ingredients, you can mix them all in a bowl and eat them. You don't need to include the liquid portion of the smoothie, but feel free to have as much of the other ingredients as you like. Don't worry, you still get the benefits of the ingredients even if they're not blended.

Snack 1

Choose one of the following for your snack. You can always have 2 tablespoons of a low-calorie balsamic vinaigrette or 3 tablespoons of a low-calorie natural hummus to dip your snack in for flavor.

15 baby carrot sticks
1 celery stalk cut into slices
15 cucumber slices
20 almonds
10 cherry tomatoes
Any piece of fruit
1 cup of any type of berries

Shake

In a perfect world, you would make your own shake using one of the recipes from chapter 7. I created these recipes with the program's cleansing goals in sharp focus. However, if you need to purchase the shakes, make sure they are 300 calories or less, contain natural ingredients, and don't contain added sugars or other artificial sweeteners and synthetic chemicals. You can add protein powder to your shake, but be mindful that they can add a lot of calories.

Clean Salad or Roasted Vegetables

Your salad should be made of 3 cups or less of leafy greens. You can include all or none of the following: 1 small tomato cut into slices (or 6 cherry tomatoes); 3 olives (any variety); 8 slices of cucumbers or the diced equivalent; 3 slices of onion; ¼ cup of diced red, green, or yellow pepper; ½ cup of shredded carrot. You're allowed to have 2 tablespoons of fat-free or low-fat dressing. Make sure the dressing you choose is 70 calories or less per 2 tablespoons, with a sodium content of 400 milligrams or less per 2 tablespoons. You can also make your own salad dressing very easily. Check out the simple recipes in the Appendix.

Instead of a salad, you can choose to have 2 cups or less of roasted vegetables. Your vegetables can include peppers, onions, Brussels sprouts, carrots, tomatoes, squash, zucchini, potatoes (sweet or white), beets, broccoli, mushrooms, and kale or other leafy greens. For cooking and seasoning you can use a tablespoon of olive oil, and salt and pepper and other herbs, to taste.

Evening Smoothie

Choose a smoothie from chapter 7 to make yourself. If you're unable to make the smoothie and must purchase it, please make sure the smoothie is 300 calories or less and that it doesn't contain added sugar. One-half teaspoon of raw organic honey is allowed if you really need it to sweeten the taste.

Snack 2

Choose one of the following for your snack. You can always have 2 tablespoons of a low-calorie balsamic vinaigrette or 3 tablespoons of a low-calorie natural hummus to dip your snack in for flavor.

15 baby carrot sticks
1 celery stalk cut into slices

15 cucumber slices
20 almonds
10 cherry tomatoes
Any piece of fruit
1 cup of any type of berries

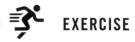 **EXERCISE**

Minimum: 30 minutes. If you want to do a little more, all the better.

You can do either the SHRED 27 Burn workout or the SHRED 15 Burn workout or choose a combination of the items below to fulfill your exercise requirement of 30 minutes. Check out the SHRED workout videos at www.shredlife.com.

15 minutes walking/running on treadmill

15 minutes on elliptical machine

15 minutes walking/jogging outside

15 minutes swimming laps

15 minutes on stationary or mobile bicycle

15 minutes on rowing machine

15 minutes of spinning class

15 minutes of Zumba

15 minutes on stair climber

15 minutes of treadmill intervals (fast walk/jog alternating with slow walk/slow jog)

225 jump rope revolutions

15 minutes of any other high-intensity cardio

JOURNAL ENTRY WEEK 1, DAY 5

What Went Well?

_____

_____

_____

What Didn't Go Well?

_____

_____

_____

What Did You Feel Throughout the Day Emotionally and Physically?

_____

_____

_____

Goals You Met Today

_____

_____

_____

Today's Inspiration

_____

_____

_____

SHRED POWER CLEANSE WEEK 1, DAY 6

SHRED THOUGHT: *Minimizing distractions means maximizing focus.* You must put distractions where they belong—in the background—and keep your mission in the foreground. There will be all types of temptations and people who will doubt, ridicule, or tease your mission, and you must be strong and remind yourself of your purpose. Distractions will tear at the edges of your focus. You truly have the strength to accomplish whatever you want. Stand up to these challenges and be stronger for it.

TODAY'S SHRED POWER CLEANSE

Morning Smoothie

Choose a smoothie from chapter 7 to make yourself. If you're unable to make the smoothie and must purchase it, make sure the smoothie is fresh (meaning it is made by the retailer with fresh ingredients) and not pre-packaged, contains 300 calories or less, and doesn't contain added sugar. One-half teaspoon of raw organic honey is allowed if you really need it to sweeten the taste.

You can also have a "deconstructed" smoothie. Instead of blending the ingredients, you can mix them all in a bowl and eat them. You don't need to include the liquid portion of the smoothie, but feel free

to have as much of the other ingredients as you like. Don't worry, you still get the benefits of the ingredients even if they're not blended.

Snack 1

Choose one of the following for your snack:

15 baby carrot sticks
1 celery stalk cut into slices
15 cucumber slices
20 almonds
10 cherry tomatoes
Any piece of fruit
1 cup of any type of berries

Shake

In a perfect world, you will make your own shake using one of the recipes from chapter 7. I created these recipes with the program's cleansing goals in sharp focus. However, if you need to purchase a shake, make sure it is 300 calories or less, contains natural ingredients, and doesn't contain added sugars or other artificial sweeteners or synthetic chemicals. You can add protein powder to your shake, but be mindful that protein powders can add a lot of calories.

Clean Salad

Your salad should be made of 3 cups or less of leafy greens. You can include all or none of the following: 1 small tomato cut into slices (or 6 cherry tomatoes); 3 olives (any variety); 8 slices of cucumbers or the diced equivalent; 3 slices of onion; ¼ cup of diced red, green, or yellow pepper; ½ cup of shredded carrot. You're allowed to have 2 tablespoons of fat-free or low-fat dressing. Make sure the dressing you choose is 70 calories or less per 2 tablespoons, with a sodium content of 400 milligrams or less per 2 tablespoons. You can also make your own salad dressing very easily. Check out the simple recipes in the Appendix.

Evening Smoothie

Choose a smoothie from chapter 7 to make yourself. If you're unable to make the smoothie and must purchase it, make sure the smoothie is fresh (meaning it is made by the retailer with fresh ingredients) and not pre-packaged, contains 300 calories or less, and doesn't contain added sugar. One-half teaspoon of raw organic honey is allowed if you really need it to sweeten the taste.

You can also have a "deconstructed" smoothie. Instead of blending the ingredients, you can mix them all in a bowl and eat them. You don't need to include the liquid portion of the smoothie, but feel free to have as much of the other ingredients as you like. Don't worry, you still get the benefits of the ingredients even if they're not blended.

Snack 2

Choose one of the following for your snack. You can always have 2 tablespoons of a low-calorie balsamic vinaigrette or 3 tablespoons of a low-calorie natural hummus to dip your snack in for flavor.

15 baby carrot sticks
1 celery stalk cut into slices
15 cucumber slices
20 almonds
10 cherry tomatoes
Any piece of fruit
1 cup of any type of berries

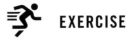

Minimum: 45 minutes. If you want to do a little more, all the better.

You can do either the SHRED 27 Burn workout or the SHRED 15 Burn workout or choose a combination of the items below to fulfill your exercise requirement of 45 minutes. Check out the SHRED workout videos at www.shredlife.com.

15 minutes walking/running on treadmill

15 minutes on elliptical machine

15 minutes walking/jogging outside

15 minutes swimming laps

15 minutes on stationary or mobile bicycle

15 minutes on rowing machine

15 minutes of spinning class

15 minutes of Zumba

15 minutes on stair climber

15 minutes of treadmill intervals (fast walk/jog alternating with slow walk/slow jog)

225 jump rope revolutions

15 minutes of any other high-intensity cardio

JOURNAL ENTRY WEEK 1, DAY 6

What Went Well?

_____

_____

_____

What Didn't Go Well?

_____

_____

_____

What Did You Feel Throughout the Day Emotionally and Physically?

_____

_____

_____

Goals You Met Today

_____

_____

_____

Today's Inspiration

_____

_____

_____

SHRED THOUGHT: *Bad habits are often not easy to break, but they are far from unbreakable.* When it comes to poor nutrition and exercise choices, changing a habit can be really difficult. But one beauty of our bodies is that they are extremely resilient. By eating better and improving your physical activity, you can reverse a lot of the accumulated damage that poor behavioral choices have caused. Just because you may not have been at your best in the past doesn't mean you can't be at your best in the future.

TODAY'S SHRED POWER CLEANSE

Morning Smoothie

Choose a smoothie from chapter 7 to make yourself. If you're unable to make the smoothie and must purchase it, make sure the smoothie is fresh (meaning it is made by the retailer with fresh ingredients) and not pre-packaged, contains 300 calories or less, and doesn't contain added sugar. One-half teaspoon of raw organic honey is allowed if you really need it to sweeten the taste.

You can also have a "deconstructed" smoothie. Instead of blending the ingredients, you can mix them all in a bowl and eat them. You don't need to include the liquid portion of the smoothie, but feel free

to have as much of the other ingredients as you like. Don't worry, you still get the benefits of the ingredients even if they're not blended.

Snack 1

Choose one of the following for your snack:

15 baby carrot sticks
1 celery stalk cut into slices
15 cucumber slices
20 almonds
10 cherry tomatoes
Any piece of fruit
1 cup of any type of berries

Shake

In a perfect world, you will make your own shake using one of the recipes from chapter 7. I created these recipes with the program's cleansing goals in sharp focus. However, if you need to purchase a shake, make sure it is 300 calories or less, contains natural ingredients, and doesn't contain added sugars or other artificial sweeteners or synthetic chemicals. You can add protein powder to your shake, but be mindful that protein powders can add a lot of calories.

Clean Salad or Roasted Vegetables

Your salad should be made of 3 cups or less of leafy greens. You can include all or none of the following: 1 small tomato cut into slices (or 6 cherry tomatoes); 3 olives (any variety); 8 slices of cucumbers or the diced equivalent; 3 slices of onion; ¼ cup of diced red, green, or yellow pepper; ½ cup of shredded carrot. You're allowed to have 2 tablespoons of fat-free or low-fat dressing. Make sure the dressing you choose is 70 calories or less per 2 tablespoons, with a sodium content of 400 milligrams or less per 2 tablespoons. You can also make your own salad dressing very easily. Check out the simple recipes in the Appendix.

Instead of a salad, you can choose to have 2 cups or less of roasted vegetables. Your vegetables can include peppers, onions, Brussels sprouts, carrots, tomatoes, squash, zucchini, potatoes (sweet or white), beets, broccoli, mushrooms, and kale or other leafy greens. For cooking and seasoning you can use a tablespoon of olive oil, and salt and pepper and other herbs, to taste.

Evening Smoothie

Choose a smoothie from chapter 7 to make yourself. If you're unable to make the smoothie and must purchase it, make sure the smoothie is fresh (meaning it is made by the retailer with fresh ingredients) and not pre-packaged, contains 300 calories or less, and doesn't contain added sugar. One-half teaspoon of raw organic honey is allowed if you really need it to sweeten the taste.

You can also have a "deconstructed" smoothie. Instead of blending the ingredients, you can mix them all in a bowl and eat them. You don't need to include the liquid portion of the smoothie, but feel free to have as much of the other ingredients as you like. Don't worry, you still get the benefits of the ingredients even if they're not blended.

Snack 2

Choose one of the following for your snack. You can always have 2 tablespoons of a low-calorie balsamic vinaigrette or 3 tablespoons of a low-calorie natural hummus to dip your snack in for flavor.

15 baby carrot sticks
1 celery stalk cut into slices
15 cucumber slices
20 almonds

10 cherry tomatoes

Any piece of fruit

1 cup of any type of berries

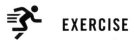 **EXERCISE**

Rest Day: Your body needs to recover in order to improve. Take this day to allow restoration.

JOURNAL ENTRY WEEK 1, DAY 7

What Went Well?

_____

_____

_____

What Didn't Go Well?

_____

_____

_____

What Did You Feel Throughout the Day Emotionally and Physically?

_____

_____

_____

Goals You Met Today

_____

_____

_____

Today's Inspiration

_____

_____

_____

5

WEEK 2: ORBIT

You have now completed one week of your two-week SHRED Power Cleanse. Your body has undergone a metamorphosis that you have likely felt in your weight, your appearance, and your energy levels. Your taste buds also have started to undergo a transformation. Foods that you might have missed and craved in the early days of the program are no longer at the top of your mind. You are nicely adapting to a cleaner way of eating, and physiologically your body is enjoying this improved environment.

Now that you are familiar with the program, this second week should come easier: you're in a groove! Most of the tough adjustments have already been made, and you have probably even found strategies that help you customize parts of the program that work best for you. Remember that no one is perfect, and perfection is not expected of you at any point in the program. The expectation is that you give it your all and do your best to make better decisions and give your body a rest from ingesting toxins and chemicals.

It's important to reiterate the importance of exercise in this program and the role it plays in helping your body undergo a complete cleanse. There are specific recommendations for the amount of time you should exercise each day (except the rest days). Do as much of what is suggested as you can, and if necessary break it up into two sessions. If you don't hit all of the exercise bench marks, that doesn't mean you will not successfully cleanse. Our goal is to increase blood flow, accelerate breathing to exchange good and bad gases, and get our skin in the game by sweating more. After a good round of exercise and hydration, you'll even feel cleaner.

Power Snack

Each day you are allowed an extra snack. This snack is meant to power you through the times when you really are hungry or feel the need for a jolt of energy. This snack is meant to be used ONLY if you need it. Don't just eat it because you want an extra snack. This Power Snack is available to you on any day of the program, at any time, but you're only allowed a maximum of one per day. Be smart with your Power Snack, save it for a stretch between meals or at a time between a snack and meal when you are really hungry. Try not to eat it at the same time as a designated snack or a time that's really close to your last snack. For your power snack, you must choose from the following list:

10 baby carrots (2 tablespoons of low-calorie dressing or
   3 tablespoons of a low-calorie natural hummus optional)
1 cup of cherries
10 cherry tomatoes
1 boiled egg with seasoning (sprinkle of salt allowed)
1 piece of fruit
1 cup of any type of berries
1 cup of any type of melon chunks
1 cup of plain air-popped popcorn
1½ cups of sugar snap peas

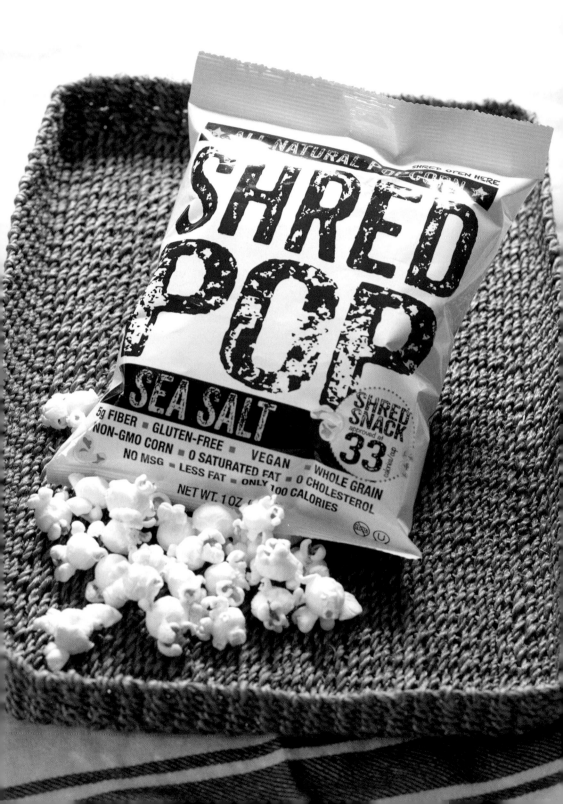

½ cup of shelled edamame beans

3 tablespoons sunflower seeds in their shells

20 almonds

1 small banana (optional: 1 tablespoon organic or natural peanut butter)

1 celery stalk (optional: 1 tablespoon organic or natural peanut butter)

Eating Schedule

The eating schedule for this week is different than week 1 so make sure you pay attention to the daily meal plan specifics. Make sure you space your meals throughout the day. Eat your first meal within an hour of getting up and your last meal no closer than 90 minutes before going to bed. Below is a sample meal schedule for someone who wakes up at 7 A.M. Your meal schedule will look different based on the time you wake up. You might not hit your eating times perfectly, and that's okay. Try your best to hit the time, but if you don't, you have a 45-minute grace period. Avoid skipping meals, but if you are 45 minutes past the time you were supposed to eat a meal or snack, then move on and don't double up on the next snack or meal because you missed the previous one. If you find yourself getting hungry later on, feel free to eat a piece of fruit.

Awake	Morning Smoothie	Snack 1	Shake	Clean Salad	Evening Smoothie	Snack 2
7 A.M.	8 A.M.	9:30 A.M.	12:00 P.M.	3:00 P.M.	6:30 P.M.	8:30 P.M.

*Don't forget your Power Snack is available to you at any time.

GUIDELINE REMINDERS

▸ All shakes and smoothies are 12 ounces (a cup and a half).

▸ All salads are fruits and veggies; only 3 tablespoons fat-free or low-fat, low-calorie clean dressing.

- ▶ Feel free to add organic protein powder (organic hemp, whey, or pea) to each shake.
- ▶ If you need to make substitutions, make smart ones that don't increase calorie counts.
- ▶ Make sure one of your smoothies is the SHRED Purple Power Detox Smoothie.
- ▶ Make sure all nuts are unsalted.
- ▶ Where the recipe calls for a specific variety of kale, you can change to a different type of your preference.
- ▶ When recipes call for frozen berries, you can substitute fresh berries, but be mindful that if you don't have ice or chilled liquid in the drink, it will be warm and needs to be refrigerated unless you don't mind room-temperature smoothies.
- ▶ Consume at least 6 cups of water each day. This should be plain flat or fizzy water, not flavored water with additives.
- ▶ You can replace the morning smoothie with a cup of whole grain cereal such as oatmeal. You can use ½ cup of low-fat, fat-free, skim, unsweetened almond, soy, or coconut milk. One-half teaspoon of raw organic honey is allowed. You can only make this replacement three times during the week.
- ▶ You can replace a smoothie, shake, or salad with a soup three times during the week, but they must be different days. You can cook your own soup or buy one. Avoid cream soups and choose broth or tomato-based soups. If you buy canned soup, go for those marked low-sodium, and make sure they contain 480 milligrams of sodium or less. The lower the sodium count the better. Acceptable soups include but are not limited to black bean, vegetable, corn, tomato, pea, butternut squash, sweet potato, lentil, chickpea, and vegetarian. These soups should be 200 calories or less.

SHRED THOUGHT: *Don't run away from something you don't want; run toward a goal.* When people want to avoid undesirable outcomes, such as a diabetes diagnosis or the need to take blood pressure medication, they often create a mind-set of running away from something they don't want to happen rather than running toward something they do want to happen. Focus not on what's behind but rather on what's out in front—your goals that pull you rather than fears that push you.

TODAY'S SHRED POWER CLEANSE

Morning Smoothie

Choose a smoothie from chapter 7 to make yourself. If you're unable to make the smoothie and must purchase it, make sure the smoothie is fresh (meaning it is made by the retailer with fresh ingredients) and not pre-packaged, contains 300 calories or less, and doesn't contain added sugar. One-half teaspoon of raw organic honey is allowed if you really need it to sweeten the taste.

You can also have a "deconstructed" smoothie. Instead of blending the ingredients, you can mix them all in a bowl and eat them. You don't need to include the liquid portion of the smoothie, but feel free to have as much of the other ingredients as you like. Don't worry, you still get the benefits of the ingredients even if they're not blended.

Snack 1

Choose one of the following for your snack. You can always have 2 tablespoons of a low-calorie balsamic vinaigrette or 3 tablespoons of a low-calorie natural hummus to dip your snack in for flavor.

8 to 10 olives (any variety)

1 cup of diced cucumber and tomato salad with 1 tablespoon of low-calorie dressing

1 cup of puffed wheat

1½ cups of sugar snap peas

3 tablespoons sunflower seeds in their shells

25 dry-roasted peanuts

17 pecans

15 cashews

30 grapes

½ cup of oven-baked kale chips

2 cups of air-popped popcorn

1 small baked sweet potato

6 raw oysters

15 baby carrot sticks

1 celery stalk cut into slices

15 cucumber slices

20 almonds

10 cherry tomatoes

Any piece of fruit

1 cup of any type of berries

Shake

In a perfect world, you will make your own shake using one of the recipes from chapter 7. I created these recipes with the program's cleansing goals in sharp focus. However, if you need to purchase the shakes, make sure they are 300 calories or less, contain natural ingredients, and don't contain added sugars or other artificial sweeteners and synthetic chemicals. You can add protein powder to your shake, but be mindful that protein powder can add a lot of calories.

Clean Salad or Roasted Vegetables

Your salad should be made of 3 cups or less of leafy greens. You can include all or none of the following: 1 small tomato cut into slices (or 6 cherry tomatoes); 3 olives (any variety); 8 slices of cucumbers or the diced equivalent; 3 slices of onion; ¼ cup of diced red, green, or yellow pepper; ½ cup of shredded carrot. You're allowed to have 2 tablespoons of fat-free or low-fat dressing. Make sure the dressing you choose is 70 calories or less per 2 tablespoons, with a sodium content of 400 milligrams or less per 2 tablespoons. You can also make your own salad dressing very easily. Check out the simple recipes in the Appendix.

Instead of a salad, you can choose to have 2 cups or less of roasted vegetables. Your vegetables can include peppers, onions, Brussels sprouts, carrots, tomatoes, squash, zucchini, potatoes (sweet or white), beets, broccoli, mushrooms, and kale or other leafy greens. For cooking and seasoning you can use a tablespoon of olive oil, and salt and pepper and other herbs, to taste.

Evening Smoothie

Choose a smoothie from chapter 7 to make yourself. If you're unable to make the smoothie and must purchase it, make sure the smoothie is 300 calories or less and that it doesn't contain added sugar. One-half teaspoon of raw organic honey is allowed if you really need it to sweeten the taste.

Snack 2

Choose one of the following for your snack. You can always have 2 tablespoons of a low-calorie balsamic vinaigrette or 3 tablespoons of a low-calorie natural hummus to dip your snack in for flavor.

8 to 10 olives (any variety)

1 cup of diced cucumber and tomato salad with 1 tablespoon of low-calorie dressing

1 cup of puffed wheat

1½ cups of sugar snap peas

3 tablespoons sunflower seeds in their shells

25 dry-roasted peanuts

17 pecans

15 cashews

20 almonds

30 grapes

½ cup raw (dehydrated) kale chips

2 cups of air-popped popcorn

1 small baked sweet potato

6 raw oysters

15 baby carrot sticks

1 celery stalk cut into slices

15 cucumber slices

10 cherry tomatoes

Any piece of fruit

1 cup of any type of berries

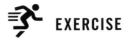

EXERCISE

Minimum: 30 minutes. If you want to do a little more, all the better.

When it comes to exercise, you get as much out of it as you put into it. Exercise is not a time to socialize and simply occupy time. It's your appointment with your body to focus on improving the way it moves, feels, and looks. One of your goals with exercise should be to push yourself to work as hard as possible in a short period of time. Remember, the time listed below is not how long you are expected to be present in an exercise environment such as the gym, rather it is meant to be how much time you are actually performing exercise. The clock doesn't start until you begin moving and it stops when you stop. While a gym can be convenient for many, you don't have to go to a gym to perform your exercise. You can do it right in your own backyard, in your bedroom, basement, or wherever you have floor space. Try to vary your workouts, so choose one that's different from the last one you did. Below you will find some 15-minute interval exercises that you might try. For example, if the program calls for 30 minutes, you can do 15 minutes of fast walking/jogging on the treadmill and 15 minutes riding the stationary or a mobile bike. You can also do 30 minutes of riding the stationary or mobile bike. But remember, regardless of what you choose, your exercise intensity is important. It's your decision how to break up the exercise, but understand that changing your routine is typically more advantageous than simply doing the same type of exercise for the entire workout.

You can do either the SHRED 27 Burn workout or the SHRED 15 Burn workout or choose a combination of the items below to fulfill your exercise requirement of 30 minutes. Check out the SHRED workout videos at www. shredlife.com.

    15 minutes walking/running on treadmill
    15 minutes on elliptical machine
    15 minutes walking/jogging outside
    15 minutes swimming laps

15 minutes on stationary or mobile bicycle

15 minutes on rowing machine

15 minutes of spinning class

15 minutes of Zumba

15 minutes on stair climber

15 minutes of treadmill intervals (fast walk/jog alternating with slow walk/slow jog)

225 jump rope revolutions

15 minutes of any other high-intensity cardio

JOURNAL ENTRY WEEK 2, DAY 1

What Went Well?

_____

_____

_____

What Didn't Go Well?

_____

_____

_____

What Did You Feel Throughout the Day Emotionally and Physically?

_____

_____

_____

Goals You Met Today

_____

_____

_____

Today's Inspiration

_____

_____

_____

SHRED THOUGHT: *Eat clean, train dirty.* The power of movement is grossly underestimated when it comes to helping your body undergo a complete cleanse. Increasing your blood circulation, breathing, and sweating all contribute to making sure your body is able to mobilize toxic substances and either neutralize or eliminate them. When you eat and drink today, think about how clean everything is that's going into your body, free of pesticide residue, artificial chemicals such as sweeteners, and synthetic compounds. When you work out today, think about all of the toxins being eliminated through your lungs and pores and being mobilized from your blood. You can't help but feel healthier.

TODAY'S SHRED POWER CLEANSE

Morning Smoothie

Choose a smoothie from chapter 7 to make yourself. If you're unable to make the smoothie and must purchase it, make sure the smoothie is fresh (meaning it is made by the retailer with fresh ingredients) and not pre-packaged, contains 300 calories or less, and doesn't contain added sugar. One-half teaspoon of raw organic honey is allowed if you really need it to sweeten the taste.

You can also have a "deconstructed" smoothie. Instead of blending the ingredients, you can mix them all in a bowl and eat them. You don't need to include the liquid portion of the smoothie, but feel free to have as much of the other ingredients as you like. Don't worry, you still get the benefits of the ingredients even if they're not blended.

Snack 1

Choose one of the following for your snack. You can always have 2 tablespoons of a low-calorie balsamic vinaigrette or 3 tablespoons of a low-calorie natural hummus to dip your snack in for flavor.

8 to 10 olives (any variety)
1 cup of diced cucumber and tomato salad with 1 tablespoon of low-calorie dressing
1 cup of puffed wheat
1½ cups of sugar snap peas
3 tablespoons sunflower seeds in their shells
25 dry-roasted peanuts
17 pecans
15 cashews
20 almonds
30 grapes
½ cup of oven-baked kale chips
2 cups of air-popped popcorn
1 small baked sweet potato
6 raw oysters
15 baby carrot sticks
1 celery stalk cut into slices
15 cucumber slices
10 cherry tomatoes
Any piece of fruit
1 cup of any type of berries

Shake

In a perfect world, you will make your own shake using one of the recipes from chapter 7. I created these recipes with the program's cleansing goals in sharp focus. However, if you need to purchase the shakes, make sure they are 300 calories or less, contain natural ingredients, and don't contain added sugars or other artificial sweeteners and synthetic chemicals. You can add protein powder to your shake, but be mindful that protein powders can add a lot of calories.

Clean Salad

Your salad should be made of 3 cups or less of leafy greens. You can include all or none of the following: 1 small tomato cut into slices (or 6 cherry tomatoes); 3 olives (any variety); 8 slices of cucumbers or the diced equivalent; 3 slices of onion; ¼ cup of diced red, green, or yellow pepper; and ½ cup of shredded carrot. You're allowed to have 2 tablespoons of fat-free or low-fat dressing. Make sure the dressing you choose is 70 calories or less per 2 tablespoons, with a sodium content of 400 milligrams or less per 2 tablespoons. You can also make your own salad dressing very easily. Check out the simple recipes in the Appendix.

Afternoon Smoothie

Choose a smoothie from chapter 7 to make yourself. If you're unable to make the smoothie and must purchase it, make sure the smoothie is fresh (meaning it is made by the retailer with fresh ingredients) and not pre-packaged, contains 300 calories or less, and doesn't contain added sugar. One-half teaspoon of raw organic honey is allowed if you really need it to sweeten the taste.

You can also have a "deconstructed" smoothie. Instead of blending the ingredients, you can mix them all in a bowl and eat them. You don't need to include the liquid portion of the smoothie, but feel free

to have as much of the other ingredients as you like. Don't worry, you still get the benefits of the ingredients even if they're not blended.

Evening Smoothie

Choose a smoothie from chapter 7 to make yourself. If you're unable to make the smoothie and must purchase it, please make sure the smoothie is 300 calories or less and that it doesn't contain added sugar. One-half teaspoon of raw organic honey is allowed if you really need it to sweeten the taste.

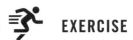 **EXERCISE**

Minimum: 30 minutes. If you want to do a little more, all the better.

You can do either the SHRED 27 Burn workout or the SHRED 15 Burn workout or choose a combination of the items below to fulfill your exercise requirement of 30 minutes. Check out the SHRED workout videos at www.shredlife.com.

- 15 minutes walking/running on treadmill
- 15 minutes on elliptical machine
- 15 minutes walking/jogging outside
- 15 minutes swimming laps
- 15 minutes on stationary or mobile bicycle
- 15 minutes on rowing machine
- 15 minutes of spinning class
- 15 minutes of Zumba
- 15 minutes on stair climber
- 15 minutes of treadmill intervals (fast walk/jog alternating with slow walk/slow jog)
- 225 jump rope revolutions
- 15 minutes of any other high-intensity cardio

JOURNAL ENTRY WEEK 2, DAY 2

What Went Well?

_____

_____

_____

What Didn't Go Well?

_____

_____

_____

What Did You Feel Throughout the Day Emotionally and Physically?

_____

_____

_____

Goals You Met Today

_____

_____

_____

Today's Inspiration

_____

_____

_____

SHRED THOUGHT: *In order to be changed, you must be challenged.* It's extremely easy to fall into a comfort zone and allow yourself to coast through life. Habits are formed, routines are established, and without even thinking you find yourself mindlessly going from one day to another, completing tasks, and accepting what life throws your way. You're sleepwalking. But if you want to change yourself, the behavior of others—or even the world—there must be a challenge. Life begins at the end of your comfort zone, so don't be afraid to push yourself, try new things, and take the path that seems more difficult. You can learn a lot of important things about yourself in moments of struggle.

TODAY'S SHRED POWER CLEANSE

Morning Smoothie

Choose a smoothie from chapter 7 to make yourself. If you're unable to make the smoothie and must purchase it, make sure the smoothie is fresh (meaning it is made by the retailer with fresh ingredients) and not pre-packaged, contains 300 calories or less, and doesn't contain added sugar. One-half teaspoon of raw organic honey is allowed if you really need it to sweeten the taste.

You can also have a "deconstructed" smoothie. Instead of blend-

ing the ingredients, you can mix them all in a bowl and eat them. You don't need to include the liquid portion of the smoothie, but feel free to have as much of the other ingredients as you like. Don't worry, you still get the benefits of the ingredients even if they're not blended.

Snack 1

Choose one of the following for your snack. You can always have 2 tablespoons of a low-calorie balsamic vinaigrette or 3 tablespoons of a low-calorie natural hummus to dip your snack in for flavor.

8 to 10 olives (any variety)

1 cup of diced cucumber and tomato salad with 1 tablespoon of low-calorie dressing

1 cup of puffed wheat

1½ cups of sugar snap peas

3 tablespoons sunflower seeds in their shells

25 dry-roasted peanuts

17 pecans

15 cashews

20 almonds

30 grapes

½ cup of oven-baked kale chips

2 cups of air-popped popcorn

1 small baked sweet potato

6 raw oysters

15 baby carrot sticks

1 celery stalk cut into slices

15 cucumber slices

10 cherry tomatoes

Any piece of fruit

1 cup of any type of berries

Afternoon Smoothie

Choose a smoothie from chapter 7 to make yourself. If you're unable to make the smoothie and must purchase it, make sure the smoothie is 300 calories or less and that it doesn't contain added sugar. One-half teaspoon of raw organic honey is allowed if you really need it to sweeten the taste.

Snack 2

Choose one of the following for your snack. You can always have 2 tablespoons of a low-calorie balsamic vinaigrette or 3 tablespoons of a low-calorie natural hummus to dip your snack in for flavor.

8 to 10 olives (any variety)

1 cup of diced cucumber and tomato salad with 1 tablespoon of low-calorie dressing

1 cup of puffed wheat

1½ cups of sugar snap peas

3 tablespoons sunflower seeds in their shells

25 dry-roasted peanuts

17 pecans

15 cashews

20 almonds

30 grapes

½ cup of raw (dehydrated) kale chips

2 cups of air-popped popcorn

1 small baked sweet potato

6 raw oysters

15 baby carrot sticks

1 celery stalk cut into slices

15 cucumber slices

10 cherry tomatoes

Any piece of fruit

1 cup of any type of berries

Clean Salad or Roasted Vegetables

Your salad should be made of 3 cups or less of leafy greens. You can include all or none of the following: 1 small tomato cut into slices (or 6 cherry tomatoes); 3 olives (any variety); 8 slices of cucumbers or the diced equivalent; 3 slices of onion; ¼ cup of diced red, green, or yellow pepper; ½ cup of shredded carrot. You're allowed to have 2 tablespoons of fat-free or low-fat dressing. Make sure the dressing you choose is 70 calories or less per 2 tablespoons, with a sodium content of 400 milligrams or less per 2 tablespoons. You can also make your own salad dressing very easily. Check out the simple recipes in the Appendix.

Instead of a salad, you can choose to have 2 cups or less of roasted vegetables. Your vegetables can include peppers, onions, Brussels sprouts, carrots, tomatoes, squash, zucchini, potatoes (sweet or white), beets, broccoli, mushrooms, and kale or other leafy greens. For cooking and seasoning you can use a tablespoon of olive oil, and salt and pepper and other herbs, to taste.

Evening Smoothie

Choose a smoothie from chapter 7 to make yourself. If you're unable to make the smoothie and must purchase it, make sure the smoothie is fresh (meaning it is made by the retailer with fresh ingredients) and not pre-packaged, contains 300 calories or less, and doesn't contain added sugar. One-half teaspoon of raw organic honey is allowed if you really need it to sweeten the taste.

You can also have a "deconstructed" smoothie. Instead of blending the ingredients, you can mix them all in a bowl and eat them. You don't need to include the liquid portion of the smoothie, but feel free to have as much of the other ingredients as you like. Don't worry, you still get the benefits of the ingredients even if they're not blended.

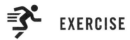 **EXERCISE**

Rest Day: Your body needs to recover in order to improve. Take this day to allow restoration.

JOURNAL ENTRY WEEK 2, DAY 3

What Went Well?

_____

_____

_____

What Didn't Go Well?

_____

_____

_____

_____

What Did You Feel Throughout the Day Emotionally and Physically?

_____

_____

_____

Goals You Met Today

_____

_____

_____

Today's Inspiration

_____

_____

SHRED THOUGHT: *Doubt is the seed of failure.* Many people lose before the game begins because they doubt their ability to win. Regardless of your chances for success, if your initial thoughts are that success is unlikely or too difficult, then these thoughts will bear fruit. Keeping yourself in a positive mind-set even when the task before you might seem Herculean in nature is a thought process that all winners share. You can be a winner, but that means you have to believe it first.

TODAY'S SHRED POWER CLEANSE

Morning Smoothie

Choose a smoothie from chapter 7 to make yourself. If you're unable to make the smoothie and must purchase it, make sure the smoothie is fresh (meaning it is made by the retailer with fresh ingredients) and not pre-packaged, contains 300 calories or less, and doesn't contain added sugar. One-half teaspoon of raw organic honey is allowed if you really need it to sweeten the taste.

You can also have a "deconstructed" smoothie. Instead of blending the ingredients, you can mix them all in a bowl and eat them. You don't need to include the liquid portion of the smoothie, but feel free

to have as much of the other ingredients as you like. Don't worry, you still get the benefits of the ingredients even if they're not blended.

Snack 1

Choose one of the following for your snack. You can always have 2 tablespoons of a low-calorie balsamic vinaigrette or 3 tablespoons of a low-calorie natural hummus to dip your snack in for flavor.

8 to 10 olives (any variety)
1 cup of diced cucumber and tomato salad with 1 tablespoon of low-calorie dressing
1 cup of puffed wheat
1½ cups of sugar snap peas
3 tablespoons sunflower seeds in their shells
25 dry-roasted peanuts
17 pecans
15 cashews
20 almonds
30 grapes
½ cup of raw (dehydrated) kale chips
2 cups of air-popped popcorn
1 small baked sweet potato
6 raw oysters
15 baby carrot sticks
1 celery stalk cut into slices
15 cucumber slices
10 cherry tomatoes
Any piece of fruit
1 cup of any type of berries

Shake

In a perfect world, you will make your own shake using one of the recipes from chapter 7. I created these recipes with the program's cleansing goals in sharp focus. However, if you need to purchase the shakes, make sure they are 300 calories or less, contain natural ingredients, and don't contain added sugars or other artificial sweeteners and synthetic chemicals. You can add protein powder to your shake, but be mindful that protein powder can add a lot of calories.

Clean Salad

Your salad should be made of 3 cups or less of leafy greens. You can include all or none of the following: 1 small tomato cut into slices (or 6 cherry tomatoes); 3 olives (any variety); 8 slices of cucumbers or the diced equivalent; 3 slices of onion; ¼ cup of diced red, green, or yellow pepper; and ½ cup of shredded carrot. You're allowed to have 2 tablespoons of fat-free or low-fat dressing. Make sure the dressing you choose is 70 calories or less per 2 tablespoons, with a sodium content of 400 milligrams or less per 2 tablespoons. You can also make your own salad dressing very easily. Check out the simple recipes in the Appendix.

Evening Smoothie

Choose a smoothie from chapter 7 to make yourself. If you're unable to make the smoothie and must purchase it, make sure the smoothie is fresh (meaning it is made by the retailer with fresh ingredients) and not pre-packaged, contains 300 calories or less, and doesn't contain added sugar. One-half teaspoon of raw organic honey is allowed if you really need it to sweeten the taste.

You can also have a "deconstructed" smoothie. Instead of blending the ingredients, you can mix them all in a bowl and eat them. You don't need to include the liquid portion of the smoothie, but feel free to have as much of the other ingredients as you like. Don't worry, you still get the benefits of the ingredients even if they're not blended.

Snack 2

Choose one of the following for your snack. You can always have 2 tablespoons of a low-calorie balsamic vinaigrette or 3 tablespoons of a low-calorie natural hummus to dip your snack in for flavor.

8 to 10 olives (any variety)

1 cup of diced cucumber and tomato salad with 1 tablespoon of low-calorie dressing

1 cup of puffed wheat

1½ cups of sugar snap peas

3 tablespoons sunflower seeds in their shells

25 dry-roasted peanuts

17 pecans

15 cashews

20 almonds

30 grapes

½ cup of raw (dehydrated) kale chips

2 cups of air-popped popcorn

1 small baked sweet potato

6 raw oysters

15 baby carrot sticks

1 celery stalk cut into slices

15 cucumber slices

10 cherry tomatoes

Any piece of fruit

1 cup of any type of berries

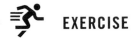 **EXERCISE**

Minimum: 30 minutes. If you want to do a little more, all the better.

You can do either the SHRED 27 Burn workout or the SHRED 15 Burn workout or choose a combination of the items below to fulfill your exercise requirement of 30 minutes. Check out the SHRED workout videos at www.shredlife.com.

15 minutes walking/running on treadmill

15 minutes on elliptical machine

15 minutes walking/jogging outside

15 minutes swimming laps

15 minutes on stationary or mobile bicycle

15 minutes on rowing machine

15 minutes of spinning class

15 minutes of Zumba

15 minutes on stair climber

15 minutes of treadmill intervals (fast walk/jog alternating with slow walk/slow jog)

225 jump rope revolutions

15 minutes of any other high-intensity cardio

JOURNAL ENTRY WEEK 2, DAY 4

What Went Well?

_____

_____

_____

What Didn't Go Well?

_____

_____

_____

What Did You Feel Throughout the Day Emotionally and Physically?

_____

_____

_____

Goals You Met Today

_____

_____

_____

Today's Inspiration

_____

_____

_____

SHRED THOUGHT: *Desire is what gets you started on a plan while habit is what keeps you going.* You started this plan because you have one or more goals you're working to achieve. Many people think about making a change but never take the first step to do it. You've taken this first step. But this plan is also about learning and establishing healthy habits. Once you adopt a new lifestyle behavior into your daily regimen, it becomes your driving force, because it's your new normal. Making a change and establishing new habits will keep you solidly planted on the road to good health and success.

TODAY'S SHRED POWER CLEANSE

Morning Smoothie

Choose a smoothie from chapter 7 to make yourself. If you're unable to make the smoothie and must purchase it, make sure the smoothie is fresh (meaning it is made by the retailer with fresh ingredients) and not pre-packaged, contains 300 calories or less, and doesn't contain added sugar. One-half teaspoon of raw organic honey is allowed if you really need it to sweeten the taste.

You can also have a "deconstructed" smoothie. Instead of blending the ingredients, you can mix them all in a bowl and eat them. You don't need to include the liquid portion of the smoothie, but feel free to have as much of the other ingredients as you like. Don't worry, you still get the benefits of the ingredients even if they're not blended.

Snack 1

Choose one of the following for your snack. You can always have 2 tablespoons of a low-calorie balsamic vinaigrette or 3 tablespoons of a low-calorie natural hummus to dip your snack in for flavor.

8 to 10 olives (any variety)
1 cup of diced cucumber and tomato salad with 1 tablespoon of
   low-calorie dressing
1 cup of puffed wheat
1½ cups of sugar snap peas
3 tablespoons sunflower seeds in their shells
25 dry-roasted peanuts
17 pecans
15 cashews
20 almonds
30 grapes
½ cup of raw (dehydrated) kale chips
2 cups of air-popped popcorn
1 small baked sweet potato
6 raw oysters
15 baby carrot sticks
1 celery stalk cut into slices
15 cucumber slices
10 cherry tomatoes
Any piece of fruit
1 cup of any type of berries

Shake

In a perfect world, you will make your own shake using one of the recipes from chapter 7. I created these recipes with the program's cleansing goals in sharp focus. However, if you need to purchase the shakes, make sure they are 300 calories or less, contain natural ingredients, and don't contain added sugars or other artificial sweeteners and synthetic chemicals. You can add protein powder to your shake, but be mindful that protein powders can add a lot of calories.

Clean Salad

Your salad should be made of 3 cups or less of leafy greens. You can include all or none of the following: 1 small tomato cut into slices (or 6 cherry tomatoes); 3 olives (any variety); 8 slices of cucumbers or the diced equivalent; 3 slices of onion; ¼ cup of diced red, green, or yellow pepper; and ½ cup of shredded carrot. You're allowed to have 2 tablespoons of fat-free or low-fat dressing. Make sure the dressing you choose is 70 calories or less per 2 tablespoons with a sodium content of 400 milligrams or less per 2 tablespoons. You can also make your own salad dressing very easily. Check out the simple recipes in the Appendix.

Evening Smoothie

Choose a smoothie from chapter 7 to make yourself. If you're unable to make the smoothie and must purchase it, make sure the smoothie is fresh (meaning it is made by the retailer with fresh ingredients) and not pre-packaged, contains 300 calories or less, and doesn't contain added sugar. One-half teaspoon of raw organic honey is allowed if you really need it to sweeten the taste.

You can also have a "deconstructed" smoothie. Instead of blending the ingredients, you can mix them all in a bowl and eat them. You don't need to include the liquid portion of the smoothie, but feel free to have as much of the other ingredients as you like. Don't worry, you still get the benefits of the ingredients even if they're not blended.

Choose one of the following for your snack. You can always have 2 tablespoons of a low-calorie balsamic vinaigrette or 3 tablespoons of a low-calorie natural hummus to dip your snack in for flavor.

    8 to 10 olives (any variety)
    1 cup of diced cucumber and tomato salad with 1 tablespoon of
        low-calorie dressing
    1 cup of puffed wheat
    1½ cups of sugar snap peas
    3 tablespoons sunflower seeds in their shells
    25 dry-roasted peanuts
    17 pecans
    15 cashews
    20 almonds
    30 grapes
    ½ cup of raw (dehydrated) kale chips
    2 cups of air-popped popcorn
    1 small baked sweet potato
    6 raw oysters
    15 baby carrot sticks
    1 celery stalk cut into slices
    15 cucumber slices
    10 cherry tomatoes
    Any piece of fruit
    1 cup of any type of berries

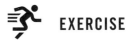 **EXERCISE**

Rest Day: Your body needs to recover in order to improve. Take this day to allow restoration.

JOURNAL ENTRY WEEK 2, DAY 5

What Went Well?

_____

_____

_____

What Didn't Go Well?

_____

_____

_____

What Did You Feel Throughout the Day Emotionally and Physically?

_____

_____

_____

Goals You Met Today

_____

_____

_____

Today's Inspiration

_____

_____

_____

SHRED POWER CLEANSE WEEK 2, DAY 6

SHRED THOUGHT: *An effort that is less than optimal is 100 percent better than no effort at all.* As the great philosopher Voltaire said, "Don't let perfect be the enemy of the good." Making an effort definitely counts for something. If you attempt to make a change and improve, you have a chance of accomplishing your goals. But if you only talk or think about what you need to do, you are guaranteeing that nothing will change and you will be no closer to your goal. Often we are so focused on perfection that we leave no room to appreciate all of the good we can achieve even if perfection isn't reached. Giving our best is the most that we can ask of ourselves.

TODAY'S SHRED POWER CLEANSE

Morning Smoothie

Choose a smoothie from chapter 7 to make yourself. If you're unable to make the smoothie and must purchase it, make sure the smoothie is fresh (meaning it is made by the retailer with fresh ingredients) and not pre-packaged, contains 300 calories or less, and doesn't contain added sugar. One-half teaspoon of raw organic honey is allowed if you really need it to sweeten the taste.

You can also have a "deconstructed" smoothie. Instead of blend-

ing the ingredients, you can mix them all in a bowl and eat them. You don't need to include the liquid portion of the smoothie, but feel free to have as much of the other ingredients as you like. Don't worry, you still get the benefits of the ingredients even if they're not blended.

Snack 1

Choose one of the following for your snack. You can always have 2 tablespoons of a low-calorie balsamic vinaigrette or 3 tablespoons of a low-calorie natural hummus to dip your snack in for flavor.

8 to 10 olives (any variety)

1 cup of diced cucumber and tomato salad with 1 tablespoon of low-calorie dressing

1 cup of puffed wheat

1½ cups of sugar snap peas

3 tablespoons sunflower seeds in their shells

25 dry-roasted peanuts

17 pecans

15 cashews

20 almonds

30 grapes

½ cup of raw (dehydrated) kale chips

2 cups of air-popped popcorn

1 small baked sweet potato

6 raw oysters

15 baby carrot sticks

1 celery stalk cut into slices

15 cucumber slices

10 cherry tomatoes

Any piece of fruit

1 cup of any type of berries

Shake

In a perfect world, you will make your own shake using one of the recipes from chapter 7. I created these recipes with the program's cleansing goals in sharp focus. However, if you need to purchase the shakes, make sure they are 300 calories or less, contain natural ingredients, and don't contain added sugars or other artificial sweeteners and synthetic chemicals. You can add protein powder to your shake, but be mindful that protein powders can add a lot of calories.

Clean Salad or Roasted Vegetables

Your salad should be made of 3 cups or less of leafy greens. You can include all or none of the following: 1 small tomato cut into slices (or 6 cherry tomatoes); 3 olives (any variety); 8 slices of cucumbers or the diced equivalent; 3 slices of onion; ¼ cup of diced red, green, or yellow pepper; ½ cup of shredded carrot. You're allowed to have 2 tablespoons of fat-free or low-fat dressing. Make sure the dressing you choose is 70 calories or less per 2 tablespoons, with a sodium content of 400 milligrams or less per 2 tablespoons. You can also make your own salad dressing very easily. Check out the simple recipes in the Appendix.

Instead of a salad, you can choose to have 2 cups or less of roasted vegetables. Your vegetables can include peppers, onions, Brussels sprouts, carrots, tomatoes, squash, zucchini, potatoes (sweet or white), beets, broccoli, mushrooms, and kale or other leafy greens. For cooking and seasoning you can use a tablespoon of olive oil, and salt and pepper and other herbs, to taste.

Evening Smoothie

Choose a smoothie from chapter 7 to make yourself. If you're unable to make the smoothie and must purchase it, make sure the smoothie is fresh (meaning it is made by the retailer with fresh ingredients) and not pre-packaged, contains 300 calories or less, and doesn't contain

added sugar. One-half teaspoon of raw organic honey is allowed if you really need it to sweeten the taste.

You can also have a "deconstructed" smoothie. Instead of blending the ingredients, you can mix them all in a bowl and eat them. You don't need to include the liquid portion of the smoothie, but feel free to have as much of the other ingredients as you like. Don't worry, you still get the benefits of the ingredients even if they're not blended.

Snack 2

Choose one of the following for your snack. You can always have 2 tablespoons of a low-calorie balsamic vinaigrette or 3 tablespoons of a low-calorie natural hummus to dip your snack in for flavor.

8 to 10 olives (any variety)

1 cup of diced cucumber and tomato salad with 1 tablespoon of low-calorie dressing

1 cup of puffed wheat

1½ cups of sugar snap peas

3 tablespoons sunflower seeds in their shells

25 dry-roasted peanuts

17 pecans

15 cashews

20 almonds

30 grapes

½ cup of raw (dehydrated) kale chips

2 cups of air-popped popcorn

1 small baked sweet potato

6 raw oysters

15 baby carrot sticks

1 celery stalk cut into slices

15 cucumber slices

10 cherry tomatoes

Any piece of fruit

1 cup of any type of berries

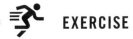 **EXERCISE**

Minimum: 30 minutes. If you want to do a little more, all the better.

You can do either the SHRED 27 Burn workout or the SHRED 15 Burn workout or choose a combination of the items below to fulfill your exercise requirement of 30 minutes. Check out the SHRED workout videos at www.shredlife.com.

15 minutes walking/running on treadmill

15 minutes on elliptical machine

15 minutes walking/jogging outside

15 minutes swimming laps

15 minutes on stationary or mobile bicycle

15 minutes on rowing machine

15 minutes of spinning class

15 minutes of Zumba

15 minutes on stair climber

15 minutes of treadmill intervals (fast walk/jog alternating with slow walk/slow jog)

225 jump rope revolutions

15 minutes of any other high-intensity cardio

JOURNAL ENTRY WEEK 2, DAY 6

What Went Well?

_____

_____

_____

What Didn't Go Well?

_____

_____

_____

What Did You Feel Throughout the Day Emotionally and Physically?

_____

_____

_____

Goals You Met Today

_____

_____

_____

Today's Inspiration

_____

_____

_____

SHRED POWER CLEANSE WEEK 2, DAY 7

SHRED THOUGHT: *Junk food can be gratifying for a few minutes, but eating clean can satisfy you for a lifetime.* Now that you're on the last day of the cleanse, look back at your journal entries and think about all of the junk foods like chips and soda and donuts that you avoided. It's quite possible you started the SHRED Power Cleanse thinking that you might never be able to go two weeks without some of these "fun foods" that are such a regular part of your diet. But look what you've been able to accomplish through focus and determination. Sure, you might've missed the taste and that temporary satisfying feeling, but the fuel you've been putting into your body the last couple of weeks has brought you so many more improvements that can last a lifetime.

TODAY'S SHRED POWER CLEANSE

Morning Smoothie

Choose a smoothie from chapter 7 to make yourself. If you're unable to make the smoothie and must purchase it, make sure the smoothie is fresh (meaning it is made by the retailer with fresh ingredients) and not pre-packaged, contains 300 calories or less, and doesn't contain added sugar. One-half teaspoon of raw organic honey is allowed if you really need it to sweeten the taste.

You can also have a "deconstructed" smoothie. Instead of blending the ingredients, you can mix them all in a bowl and eat them. You don't need to include the liquid portion of the smoothie, but feel free to have as much of the other ingredients as you like. Don't worry, you still get the benefits of the ingredients even if they're not blended.

Snack 1

Choose one of the following for your snack. You can always have 2 tablespoons of a low-calorie balsamic vinaigrette or 3 tablespoons of a low-calorie natural hummus to dip your snack in for flavor.

8 to 10 olives (any variety)
1 cup of diced cucumber and tomato salad with 1 tablespoon of
    low-calorie dressing
1 cup of puffed wheat
1½ cups of sugar snap peas
3 tablespoons sunflower seeds in their shells
25 dry-roasted peanuts
17 pecans
15 cashews
20 almonds
30 grapes
½ cup of raw (dehydrated) kale chips
2 cups of air-popped popcorn
1 small baked sweet potato
6 raw oysters
15 baby carrot sticks
1 celery stalk cut into slices
15 cucumber slices
10 cherry tomatoes
Any piece of fruit
1 cup of any type of berries

Shake

In a perfect world, you will make your own shake using one of the recipes from chapter 7. I created these recipes with the program's cleansing goals in sharp focus. However, if you need to purchase the shakes, make sure they are 300 calories or less, contain natural ingredients, and don't contain added sugars or other artificial sweeteners and synthetic chemicals. You can add protein powder to your shake, but be mindful that protein powder can add a lot of calories.

Clean Salad or Roasted Vegetables

Your salad should be made of 3 cups or less of leafy greens. You can include all or none of the following: 1 small tomato cut into slices (or 6 cherry tomatoes); 3 olives (any variety); 8 slices of cucumbers or the diced equivalent; 3 slices of onion; ¼ cup of diced red, green, or yellow pepper; ½ cup of shredded carrot. You're allowed to have 2 tablespoons of fat-free or low-fat dressing. Make sure the dressing you choose is 70 calories or less per 2 tablespoons, with a sodium content of 400 milligrams or less per 2 tablespoons. You can also make your own salad dressing very easily. Check out the simple recipes in the Appendix.

Instead of a salad, you can choose to have 2 cups or less of roasted vegetables. Your vegetables can include peppers, onions, Brussels sprouts, carrots, tomatoes, squash, zucchini, potatoes (sweet or white), beets, broccoli, mushrooms, and kale or other leafy greens. For cooking and seasoning you can use a tablespoon of olive oil, and salt and pepper and other herbs, to taste.

Evening Smoothie

Choose a smoothie from chapter 7 to make yourself. If you're unable to make the smoothie and must purchase it, make sure the smoothie is fresh (meaning it is made by the retailer with fresh ingredients) and not pre-packaged, contains 300 calories or less, and doesn't contain

added sugar. One-half teaspoon of raw organic honey is allowed if you really need it to sweeten the taste.

You can also have a "deconstructed" smoothie. Instead of blending the ingredients, you can mix them all in a bowl and eat them. You don't need to include the liquid portion of the smoothie, but feel free to have as much of the other ingredients as you like. Don't worry, you still get the benefits of the ingredients even if they're not blended.

Snack 2

Choose one of the following for your snack. You can always have 2 tablespoons of a low-calorie balsamic vinaigrette or 3 tablespoons of a low-calorie natural hummus to dip your snack in for flavor.

8 to 10 olives (any variety)

1 cup of diced cucumber and tomato salad with 1 tablespoon of low-calorie dressing

1 cup of puffed wheat

1½ cups of sugar snap peas

3 tablespoons sunflower seeds in their shells

25 dry-roasted peanuts

17 pecans

15 cashews

20 almonds

30 grapes

½ cup of raw (dehydrated) kale chips

2 cups of air-popped popcorn

1 small baked sweet potato

6 raw oysters

15 baby carrot sticks

1 celery stalk cut into slices

15 cucumber slices

10 cherry tomatoes

Any piece of fruit

1 cup of any type of berries

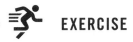 **EXERCISE**

Minimum: 30 minutes. If you want to do a little more, all the better.

While the food portion of the cleanse comes to a close with this last day, the exercise you've been doing should continue for the rest of your life. Exercise is something that is beneficial and can be enjoyed at all ages and in various forms. Whether through sports, the gym, or home activities, exercising continues to deliver breathtaking health benefits that affect everything from how fast you age to your risk for heart disease and dementia. Exercise should not be looked upon as a chore, rather an opportunity that can help you maximize all that life has to offer.

You can do either the SHRED 27 Burn workout or the SHRED 15 Burn workout or choose a combination of the items below to fulfill your exercise requirement of 30 minutes. Check out the SHRED workout videos at www. shredlife.com.

15 minutes walking/running on treadmill

15 minutes on elliptical machine

15 minutes walking/jogging outside

15 minutes swimming laps

15 minutes on stationary or mobile bicycle

15 minutes on rowing machine

15 minutes of spinning class

15 minutes of Zumba

15 minutes on stair climber

15 minutes of treadmill intervals (fast walk/jog alternating with slow walk/slow jog)

225 jump rope revolutions

15 minutes of any other high-intensity cardio

JOURNAL ENTRY WEEK 2, DAY 7

What Went Well?

_____

_____

_____

What Didn't Go Well?

_____

_____

_____

What Did You Feel Throughout the Day Emotionally and Physically?

_____

_____

_____

Goals You Met Today

_____

_____

_____

Today's Inspiration

_____

_____

_____

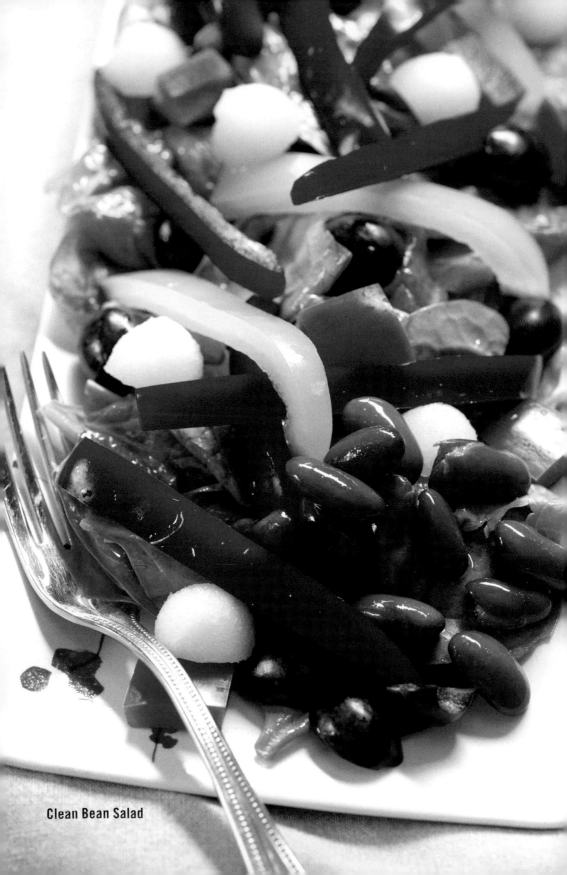

Clean Bean Salad

6

SHRED POWER WEEKEND CLEANSE

There are times when you feel like you simply need a quick reset. You might have had a week when you didn't eat or drink your best. You might be feeling sluggish or bloated. You are not alone. There are times when we all feel this way and wish we could do something about it. Well, now you can! The SHRED Power Weekend Cleanse is a three-day cleanse designed to help you push the reset button and cleanse your system of any negative effects from the previous week. The beauty of the weekend cleanse is that it's short, straightforward, gives immediate results, and you can do it as many times as you like.

One caveat about the SHRED Power Weekend Cleanse: you *must* follow it to the letter for it to be most effective. You only have three days to reset your body, and this is not a lot of time, so there is little room for deviation from the plan. You will be best served to make these meals yourself; if they are being made by someone else, make sure the ingredients are correct and the meals are prepared exactly as called for, without any additional ingredients. If you have done the two-week program, you will notice that this is a little more restrictive because of the limited time you have to achieve results. Since we are trying to maximize our body's flush of the previous weeks, there are certain things that are off-limit for these three days. Fried foods, cream sauces, bread, cakes, cookies, alcohol, chips, added sugars, red meat, and white flour products are to be avoided during this period. Our focus is clean eating, which means as little processing as possible since processing foods is what tends to add all kinds of chemicals and ingredients that don't rank very high on the healthiness scale. Even if you haven't done the two-week cleanse, you can still do this Weekend Power Cleanse.

Power Snack

Each day you are allowed an extra snack. This snack is meant to power you through the times when you really are hungry or feel the need for a jolt of energy. This snack is meant to be used ONLY if you need it. Don't just eat it because you want an extra snack. This Power Snack is available to you on any day of the program, at any time but you're only allowed a maximum of one per day. Be smart with your Power Snack, save it for a stretch between meals or at a time between a snack and meal when you are really hungry. Try not to eat it at the same time as a designated snack or a time that's really close to your last snack. For your power snack, you must choose from the following list:

10 baby carrots (2 tablespoons of low-calorie dressing
    or 3 tablespoons of a low-calorie natural hummus optional)
1 cup of cherries
10 cherry tomatoes
1 boiled egg with seasoning (sprinkle of salt allowed)
1 piece of fruit
1 cup of any type of berries
1 cup of any type of melon chunks

1 cup of plain air popped popcorn

1½ cups of sugar snap peas

½ cup of shelled edamame beans

3 tablespoons of sunflower seeds in their shells

20 almonds

1 small banana (optional: 1 tablespoon organic or natural
   peanut butter)

1 celery stalk (optional: 1 tablespoon organic or
   natural peanut butter)

GUIDELINE REMINDERS

▸ All shakes and smoothies are 12 ounces (a cup and a half).

▸ All salads are fruits and veggies; only 3 tablespoons of fat-free or low-fat low-calorie clean dressing.

▸ Feel free to add organic protein powder to each shake (organic hemp, whey, or pea).

▸ If you need to make substitutions, make smart ones that don't increase calorie counts.

▸ Make sure one of your smoothies is the SHRED Purple Power Detox Smoothie.

▸ Consume at least 6 cups of water each day. This should be plain, flat, or fizzy water, not flavored water with additives.

▸ You can replace the morning smoothie with a cup of whole grain cereal such as oatmeal. You can use ½ cup of low-fat, fat-free, skim, unsweetened almond, soy, or coconut milk. One-half tea-spoon of raw organic honey is allowed. You can only make this replacement once during these three days.

SHRED WEEKEND POWER CLEANSE DAY 1

TODAY'S SHRED POWER CLEANSE

Remember, one of your smoothies should be the Purple Power Detox Smoothie.

Below is a sample schedule of what your day might look like. Alter the day based on your own day's timing.

Awake	Morning Smoothie	Snack 1	Afternoon Smoothie	Snack 2	Clean Salad	Evening Smoothie
7 A.M.	8 A.M.	10:30 A.M.	12:30 P.M.	2:30 P.M.	3:30 P.M.	6:30 P.M.

*Don't forget your Power Snack is available to you at any time.

Morning Smoothie

Choose a smoothie from chapter 7 to make yourself. If you're unable to make the smoothie and must purchase it, make sure the smoothie is fresh (meaning it is made by the retailer with fresh ingredients) and not pre-packaged, contains 300 calories or less, and doesn't contain added sugar. One-half teaspoon of raw organic honey is allowed if you really need it to sweeten the taste.

You can also have a "deconstructed" smoothie. Instead of blending the ingredients, you can mix them all in a bowl and eat them. You don't need to include the liquid portion of the smoothie, but feel free to have as much of the other ingredients as you like. Don't worry, you still get the benefits of the ingredients even if they're not blended.

Snack 1

Choose one of the following for your snack. You can always have 2 tablespoons of a low-calorie balsamic vinaigrette or 3 tablespoons of a low-calorie natural hummus to dip your snack in for flavor.

8 to 10 olives (any variety)

1 cup of diced cucumber and tomato salad with 1 tablespoon of low-calorie dressing

1 cup of puffed wheat

1½ cups of sugar snap peas

3 tablespoons sunflower seeds in their shells

25 dry-roasted peanuts

17 pecans

15 cashews

20 almonds

30 grapes

½ cup of raw (dehydrated) kale chips

2 cups of air-popped popcorn

1 small baked sweet potato

6 raw oysters

15 baby carrot sticks

1 celery stalk cut into slices

15 cucumber slices

10 cherry tomatoes

Any piece of fruit

1 cup of any type of berries

Afternoon Smoothie

Choose a smoothie from chapter 7 to make yourself. If you're unable to make the smoothie and must purchase it, make sure the smoothie is fresh (meaning it is made by the retailer with fresh ingredients) and not pre-packaged, contains 300 calories or less, and doesn't contain added sugar. One-half teaspoon of raw organic honey is allowed if you really need it to sweeten the taste.

You can also have a "deconstructed" smoothie. Instead of blending the ingredients, you can mix them all in a bowl and eat them. You don't need to include the liquid portion of the smoothie, but feel free to have as much of the other ingredients as you like. Don't worry, you still get the benefits of the ingredients even if they're not blended.

Snack 2

Choose one of the following for your snack. You can always have 2 tablespoons of a low-calorie balsamic vinaigrette or 3 tablespoons of a low-calorie natural hummus to dip your snack in for flavor.

8 to 10 olives (any variety)
1 cup of diced cucumber and tomato salad with 1 tablespoon of low-calorie dressing
1 cup of puffed wheat
1½ cups of sugar snap peas
3 tablespoons sunflower seeds in their shells
25 dry-roasted peanuts
17 pecans
15 cashews
20 almonds
30 grapes
½ cup of raw (dehydrated) kale chips
2 cups of air-popped popcorn

1 small baked sweet potato

6 raw oysters

15 baby carrot sticks

1 celery stalk cut into slices

15 cucumber slices

10 cherry tomatoes

Any piece of fruit

1 cup of any type of berries

Clean Salad or Roasted Vegetables

Your salad should be made of 3 cups or less of leafy greens. You can include all or none of the following: 1 small tomato cut into slices (or 6 cherry tomatoes); 3 olives (any variety); 8 slices of cucumbers or the diced equivalent; 3 slices of onion; ¼ cup of diced red, green, or yellow pepper; ½ cup of shredded carrot. You're allowed to have 2 tablespoons of fat-free or low-fat dressing. Make sure the dressing you choose is 70 calories or less per 2 tablespoons, with a sodium content of 400 milligrams or less per 2 tablespoons. You can also make your own salad dressing very easily. Check out the simple recipes in the Appendix.

Instead of a salad, you can choose to have 2 cups or less of roasted vegetables. Your vegetables can include peppers, onions, Brussels sprouts, carrots, tomatoes, squash, zucchini, potatoes (sweet or white), beets, broccoli, mushrooms, and kale or other leafy greens. For cooking and seasoning you can use a tablespoon of olive oil, and salt and pepper and other herbs, to taste.

Evening Smoothie

Choose a smoothie from chapter 7 to make yourself. If you're unable to make the smoothie and must purchase it, make sure the smoothie is fresh (meaning it is made by the retailer with fresh ingredients) and

not pre-packaged, contains 300 calories or less, and doesn't contain added sugar. One-half teaspoon of raw organic honey is allowed if you really need it to sweeten the taste.

You can also have a "deconstructed" smoothie. Instead of blending the ingredients, you can mix them all in a bowl and eat them. You don't need to include the liquid portion of the smoothie, but feel free to have as much of the other ingredients as you like. Don't worry, you still get the benefits of the ingredients even if they're not blended.

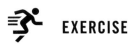 **EXERCISE**

Minimum: 45 minutes. If you want to do a little more, all the better.

When it comes to exercise, you get as much out of it as you put into it. Exercise is not a time to socialize and simply occupy time. It's your appointment with your body to focus on improving the way it moves, feels, and looks. One of your goals with exercise should be to push yourself to work as hard as possible in a short period of time. Remember, the time listed below is not how long you are expected to be present in an exercise environment such as the gym, rather it is meant to be how much time you are actually performing exercise. The clock doesn't start until you begin moving and it stops when you stop. While a gym can be convenient for many, you don't have to go to a gym to perform your exercise. You can do it right in your own backyard, in your bedroom, basement, or wherever you have floor space. Try to vary your workouts, so choose one that's different from the last one you did. Below you will find some 15-minute interval exercises that you might try. For example, if the program calls for 45 minutes, you can do 15 minutes of fast walking/jogging on the treadmill, 15 minutes riding the stationary or a mobile bike, and 15 minutes on the stair climber. You can also do 30 minutes of riding the stationary or mobile bike. But remember, regardless of what you choose, your exercise intensity is important. It's your decision how to break up the exercise, but understand that changing your routine is typically more advantageous than simply doing the same type of exercise for the entire workout.

You can do either the SHRED 27 Burn workout or the SHRED 15 Burn workout or choose a combination of the items below to fulfill your exercise requirement of 45 minutes. Check out the SHRED workout videos at www.shredlife.com.

15 minutes walking/running on treadmill

15 minutes on elliptical machine

15 minutes walking/jogging outside

15 minutes swimming laps

15 minutes on stationary or mobile bicycle

15 minutes on rowing machine

15 minutes of spinning class

15 minutes of Zumba

15 minutes on stair climber

15 minutes of treadmill intervals (fast walk/jog alternating with slow walk/slow jog)

225 jump rope revolutions

15 minutes of any other high-intensity cardio

SHRED WEEKEND POWER CLEANSE DAY 2

TODAY'S SHRED POWER CLEANSE:

Remember, one of your smoothies should be the Purple Power Detox Smoothie.

Below is a sample schedule of what your day might look like. Alter the day based on your own day's timing.

Awake	Morning Smoothie	Snack 1	Soup	Clean Salad	Evening Smoothie	Soup
7 A.M.	8 A.M.	9:30 A.M.	12:00 A.M.	3:00 P.M.	6:30 P.M.	8:30 P.M.

*Don't forget your Power Snack is available to you at any time.

Morning Smoothie

Choose a smoothie from chapter 7 to make yourself. If you're unable to make the smoothie and must purchase it, make sure the smoothie is fresh (meaning it is made by the retailer with fresh ingredients) and not pre-packaged, contains 300 calories or less, and doesn't contain added sugar. One-half teaspoon of raw organic honey is allowed if you really need it to sweeten the taste.

You can also have a "deconstructed" smoothie. Instead of blending the ingredients, you can mix them all in a bowl and eat them. You don't need to include the liquid portion of the smoothie, but feel free to have as much of the other ingredients as you like. Don't worry, you still get the benefits of the ingredients even if they're not blended.

Snack 1

Choose one of the following for your snack. You can always have 2 tablespoons of a low-calorie balsamic vinaigrette or 3 tablespoons of a low-calorie natural hummus to dip your snack in for flavor.

8 to 10 olives (any variety)

1 cup of diced cucumber and tomato salad with 1 tablespoon of low-calorie dressing

1 cup of puffed wheat

1½ cups of sugar snap peas

3 tablespoons sunflower seeds in their shells

25 dry-roasted peanuts

17 pecans

15 cashews

20 almonds

30 grapes

½ cup of raw (dehydrated) kale chips

2 cups of air-popped popcorn

1 small baked sweet potato

6 raw oysters

15 baby carrot sticks

1 celery stalk cut into slices

15 cucumber slices

10 cherry tomatoes

Any piece of fruit

1 cup of any type of berries

Soup

You can cook your own soup or purchase one. You must be careful, however, of the ingredients so that you can keep eating as cleanly as possible. Avoid cream soups and instead choose broth or tomato-based soups. If you buy canned soup, beware of the sodium content. Go for those marked low-sodium, and make sure they contain 480 milligrams of sodium or less per serving. The lower the sodium count the better. Acceptable soups would include but are not limited to black bean, vegetable, corn, tomato, pea, butternut squash, sweet potato, lentil, chickpea, and vegetarian. These soups should also be 200 calories or less.

Clean Salad or Roasted Vegetables

Your salad should be made of 3 cups or less of leafy greens. You can include all or none of the following: 1 small tomato cut into slices (or 6 cherry tomatoes); 3 olives (any variety); 8 slices of cucumbers or the diced equivalent; 3 slices of onion; ¼ cup of diced red, green, or yellow pepper; ½ cup of shredded carrot. You're allowed to have 2 tablespoons of fat-free or low-fat dressing. Make sure the dressing you choose is 70 calories or less per 2 tablespoons, with a sodium content of 400 milligrams or less per 2 tablespoons. You can also make your own salad dressing very easily. Check out the simple recipes in the Appendix.

Instead of a salad, you can choose to have 2 cups or less of roasted vegetables. Your vegetables can include peppers, onions, Brussels sprouts, carrots, tomatoes, squash, zucchini, potatoes (sweet or white), beets, broccoli, mushrooms, and kale or other leafy greens. For cooking and seasoning you can use a tablespoon of olive oil, and salt and pepper and other herbs, to taste.

Evening Smoothie

Choose a smoothie from chapter 7 to make yourself. If you're unable to make the smoothie and must purchase it, make sure the smoothie is fresh (meaning it is made by the retailer with fresh ingredients) and not pre-packaged, contains 300 calories or less, and doesn't contain added sugar. One-half teaspoon of raw organic honey is allowed if you really need it to sweeten the taste.

You can also have a "deconstructed" smoothie. Instead of blending the ingredients, you can mix them all in a bowl and eat them. You don't need to include the liquid portion of the smoothie, but feel free

to have as much of the other ingredients as you like. Don't worry, you still get the benefits of the ingredients even if they're not blended.

Soup

You can cook your own soup or purchase one. You must be careful, however, of the ingredients so that you can keep eating as cleanly as possible. Avoid cream soups and choose broth or tomato-based soups. If you buy canned soup, beware of the sodium content. Go for those marked low-sodium, and make sure they contain 480 milligrams of sodium or less per serving. The lower the sodium count the better. Acceptable soups would include but are not limited to black bean, vegetable, corn, tomato, pea, butternut squash, sweet potato, lentil, chickpea, and vegetarian. These soups should also be 200 calories or less.

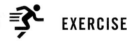 **EXERCISE**

Minimum: 30 minutes. If you want to do a little more, all the better.

You can do either the SHRED 27 Burn workout or the SHRED 15 Burn workout or choose a combination of the items below to fulfill your exercise requirement of 30 minutes. Check out the SHRED workout videos at www.shredlife.com.

- 15 minutes walking/running on treadmill
- 15 minutes on elliptical machine
- 15 minutes walking/jogging outside
- 15 minutes swimming laps
- 15 minutes on stationary or mobile bicycle
- 15 minutes on rowing machine
- 15 minutes of spinning class
- 15 minutes of Zumba
- 15 minutes on stair climber
- 15 minutes of treadmill intervals (fast walk/jog alternating with slow walk/slow jog)
- 225 jump rope revolutions
- 15 minutes of any other high-intensity cardio

SHRED WEEKEND POWER CLEANSE DAY 3

TODAY'S SHRED POWER CLEANSE

Remember, one of your smoothies should be the Purple Power Detox Smoothie.

Below is a sample schedule of what your day might look like. Alter the day based on your own day's timing.

Awake	Morning Shake	Snack 1	Clean Salad	Soup	Evening Smoothie	Snack 2
7 A.M.	8 A.M.	10:00 A.M.	12:00 P.M.	3:00 P.M.	6:30 P.M.	8:00 P.M.

*Don't forget your Power Snack is available to you at any time.

Morning Shake

In a perfect world, you will make your own shake using one of the recipes from chapter 7. I created these recipes with the program's cleansing goals in sharp focus. However, if you need to purchase a shake, make sure it is fresh (meaning it is made by the retailer with fresh ingredients) and not pre-packaged, contains 300 calories or less, contains natural ingredients, and doesn't contain added sugars or other artificial sweeteners or synthetic chemicals. You can add organic protein powder to your shake, but be mindful that protein powders can add a lot of calories so take that into consideration.

Snack 1

Choose one of the following for your snack. You can always have 2 tablespoons of a low-calorie balsamic vinaigrette or 3 tablespoons of a low-calorie natural hummus to dip your snack in for flavor.

8 to 10 olives (any variety)

1 cup of diced cucumber and tomato salad with 1 tablespoon of
   low-calorie dressing

1 cup of puffed wheat

1½ cups of sugar snap peas

3 tablespoons sunflower seeds in their shells

25 dry-roasted peanuts

17 pecans

15 cashews

20 almonds

30 grapes

½ cup of raw (dehydrated) kale chips

2 cups of air-popped popcorn

1 small baked sweet potato

6 raw oysters

15 baby carrot sticks

1 celery stalk cut into slices

15 cucumber slices

10 cherry tomatoes

Any piece of fruit

1 cup of any type of berries

Clean Salad or Roasted Vegetables

Your salad should be made of 3 cups or less of leafy greens. You can include all or none of the following: 1 small tomato cut into slices (or 6 cherry tomatoes); 3 olives (any variety); 8 slices of cucumbers or the diced equivalent; 3 slices of onion; ¼ cup of diced red, green, or yellow pepper; ½ cup of shredded carrot. You're allowed to have 2 tablespoons of fat-free or low-fat dressing. Make sure the dressing you choose is 70 calories or less per 2 tablespoons, with a sodium content of 400 milligrams or less per 2 tablespoons. You can also make your own salad dressing very easily. Check out the simple recipes in the Appendix.

Instead of a salad, you can choose to have 2 cups or less of roasted vegetables. Your vegetables can include peppers, onions, Brussels sprouts, carrots, tomatoes, squash, zucchini, potatoes (sweet or white), beets, broccoli, mushrooms, and kale or other leafy greens. For cooking and seasoning you can use a tablespoon of olive oil, and salt and pepper and other herbs, to taste.

Soup

You can cook your own soup or purchase one. You must be careful, however, of the ingredients so that you can keep eating as cleanly as possible. Avoid cream soups and choose broth or tomato-based soups. If you buy canned soup, beware of the sodium content. Go for those marked low-sodium, and make sure they contain 480 milligrams of sodium or less per serving. The lower the sodium count the better. Acceptable soups would include but are not limited to black bean, vegetable, corn, tomato, pea, butternut squash, sweet potato, lentil, chickpea, and vegetarian. These soups should also be 200 calories or less.

Evening Smoothie

Choose a smoothie from chapter 7 to make yourself. If you're unable to make the smoothie and must purchase it, make sure the smoothie is fresh (meaning it is made by the retailer with fresh ingredients) and not pre-packaged, contains 300 calories or less, and doesn't contain added sugar. One-half teaspoon of raw organic honey is allowed if you really need it to sweeten the taste.

You can also have a "deconstructed" smoothie. Instead of blending the ingredients, you can mix them all in a bowl and eat them. You don't need to include the liquid portion of the smoothie, but feel free to have as much of the other ingredients as you like. Don't worry, you still get the benefits of the ingredients even if they're not blended.

Snack 2

Choose one of the following for your snack. You can always have 2 tablespoons of a low-calorie balsamic vinaigrette or 3 tablespoons of a low-calorie natural hummus to dip your snack in for flavor.

8 to 10 olives (any variety)
1 cup of diced cucumber and tomato salad with 1 tablespoon of low-calorie dressing
1 cup of puffed wheat
1½ cups of sugar snap peas
3 tablespoons sunflower seeds in their shells
25 dry-roasted peanuts
17 pecans
15 cashews
20 almonds
30 grapes
½ cup of raw (dehydrated) kale chips
2 cups of air-popped popcorn
1 small baked sweet potato

6 raw oysters

    15 baby carrot sticks

    1 celery stalk cut into slices

    15 cucumber slices

    10 cherry tomatoes

    Any piece of fruit

    1 cup of any type of berries

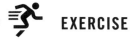 **EXERCISE**

Minimum: 30 minutes. If you want to do a little more, all the better.

You can do either the SHRED 27 Burn workout or the SHRED 15 Burn workout or choose a combination of the items below to fulfill your exercise requirement of 30 minutes. Check out the SHRED workout videos at www. shredlife.com.

15 minutes walking/running on treadmill

15 minutes on elliptical machine

15 minutes walking/jogging outside

15 minutes swimming laps

15 minutes on stationary or mobile bicycle

15 minutes on rowing machine

15 minutes of spinning class

15 minutes of Zumba

15 minutes on stair climber

15 minutes of treadmill intervals (fast walk/jog alternating with slow walk/slow jog)

225 jump rope revolutions

15 minutes of any other high-intensity cardio

7

SMOOTHIES AND SHAKES

Smoothies and shakes are a great way to get the nutrition you need at a much lower calorie price point than a standard meal. They are filled with fruits, vegetables, and other ingredients that really help your body function better, fight disease, and feel satisfied. Smoothies and shakes are also convenient because they are easy to make and carry if you're in a rush and on the go. Make them in a matter of minutes and refrigerate or freeze whatever's left over to drink at another time. They can hold up to seventy-two hours in a refrigerator and two weeks in a freezer. Make sure you blend or mix them before drinking as the ingredients tend to separate over time. These smoothies and shakes have been designed to yield two 12-ounce servings, which means you can drink up to a cup and a half for each serving.

There is enough variety here that you should find several smoothies you like. If not, take some of the recipes and make small modifications to customize for your taste. Some of the recipes include flaxseed oil. If you prefer ground flaxseed, make that substitution. This will make your drink a little seedier in texture, but you will also be adding more fiber and protein. Many of the drinks suggest added protein powder.

Be mindful that not all protein powders are alike, so choose something organic and not full of synthetic compounds.

Here are a few useful tips about making smoothies and shakes:

▶ Use cold-pressed apple juice (substitute fresh if available) for a sweeter drink.
▶ If you want to make a drink less sweet, use water instead of juice.
▶ For a thicker smoothie, use frozen fruits and add more ice.
▶ To thin your smoothie, use fresh fruit, less ice, and juice as your liquid base.
▶ For thicker shakes, use whole cow's milk, although unsweetened soy, almond, and coconut milk are acceptable substitutions.
▶ The longer you blend the ingredients, the smoother the finished product.
▶ Put the liquid in the blender first and add frozen ingredients last.
▶ Cut up produce into smaller chunks because they are easier to blend.
▶ When a recipe calls for strawberries, you can use sliced or whole strawberries. When using frozen strawberries, sliced are easier to blend.
▶ Where the recipe calls for apple juice, you can always substitute with fresh apple cider.
▶ More powerful blending will be needed when making smoothies that include the peel, seeds, and/or cores.
▶ Even if the recipe calls for peeling the fruit, you can opt to keep the peel intact. If that is the case, choose organic fruits.
▶ The riper the banana, the sweeter it is. You can freeze the banana whole or cut it into sections and freeze it that way.
▶ Where the recipe calls for flavored yogurt, if you don't have access to it or prefer plain yogurt, it's alright to make that substitution.
▶ Store smoothies in glass jars for up to 72 hours, because they keep longer and taste fresher when you go back to drink them.

THE PURPLE POWER DETOX SMOOTHIE

This is the signature drink of the SHRED Power Cleanse. The combination of the two most popular berries—strawberries and blueberries—are a flavorful start to this cleansing concoction. Blueberries, a detox super food, are packed with fiber, vitamins K and C, and manganese, and loaded with antioxidants, which are crucial for maintaining a healthy liver—the body's major detox organ. Strawberries add significant doses of vitamin C, manganese, fiber, and folate, as well as more antioxidants to help fight diseases and keep the body primed to cleanse. Flaxseed oil magnifies the drink's cleansing power by adding more fiber, which helps the gut eliminate excess toxins. Throw in a kick of fresh lemon juice to brighten the flavor and your powerful mixture is complete.

SERVINGS: 2
SERVING SIZE: 12 OZ

1 cup cold-pressed apple juice (substitute fresh if available)

1 cup frozen blueberries (fresh can be used, but if so, use 1 cup of ice cubes to make the drink immediately cold)

1 cup red Anjou pear, peeled, cored, and sliced

½ cup low-fat strawberry or plain yogurt

½ cup frozen sliced strawberries (substitute fresh if preferred)

½ cup loosely packed curly kale, stems removed

2 tablespoons unfiltered organic flaxseed oil

Juice of ½ large lemon

Combine all ingredients in a blender and purée until smooth. Drink with pleasure!

NUTRITIONAL INFORMATION PER SERVING: 300 cal., 15 g fat, 2 g sat. fat, 43 g carb., 3 g protein, 42 mg sodium, 32 g sugar, 6 g fiber.

PURPLE PANIC SMOOTHIE

This purple delight satisfies multiple senses. Delectable to the eye, sweet on the tongue, and creamy as it goes down, consuming it is a full-body experience. With 6 grams of protein, 5 grams of fiber, and extremely little in the way of fat, this drink packs it in for only 166 calories. This smoothie is an exemplar when it comes to getting as much nutrition as possible for relatively little caloric expenditure. This drink is so enjoyable, consuming one might leave you panicking to get your hands on another. No worries, the recipe makes two servings, so drink one now and save one for later.

SERVINGS: 2
SERVING SIZE: 12 OZ

1 cup unsweetened almond milk (or substitute with unsweetened soy or coconut milk)
1 cup frozen blueberries
1 cup loosely packed baby spinach, stems removed

1 ripe small banana, peeled and sliced
½ cup low-fat plain yogurt
½ cup sliced fresh strawberries (substitute frozen if fresh are not available)
½ teaspoon peeled and grated ginger

Combine all ingredients in a blender and purée until smooth. Throw it back with gusto!

NUTRITIONAL INFORMATION PER SERVING: 166 cal., 3 g fat, 1 g sat. fat, 32 g carb., 6 g protein, 131 mg sodium, 22 g sugar, 5 g fiber.

ISLAND BREEZE SMOOTHIE

Warm breezes, sandy beaches, clear blue water—you'll conjure them all with this island-inspired smoothie. Coconut, mango, and papaya—each full of flavor in its own right—are even more delectable when combined. For less than 300 calories, you get 3 grams of protein, 4 grams of fiber, and a satisfying feeling of fullness as if you've just eaten a meal. What a bargain!

SERVINGS: 2
SERVING SIZE: 12 OZ

1 cup chilled unsweetened coconut water (substitute cold-pressed apple juice for a sweeter drink)
1 cup fresh or frozen peeled mango slices
1 cup loosely packed kale, stems removed

1 ripe medium banana, peeled and sliced
½ cup peeled, seeded, and chopped fresh ripe papaya
2 tablespoons low-fat plain yogurt
2 tablespoons unfiltered organic flaxseed oil
Juice of ½ large lemon

Combine all ingredients in a blender and purée until smooth. Enjoy!

NUTRITIONAL INFORMATION PER SERVING: 272 cal., 14 g fat, 2 g sat. fat, 37 g carb., 3 g protein, 31 mg sodium, 23 g sugar, 4 g fiber.

MAMA MIA CHIA SMOOTHIE

When you hear the word *chia*, your mind probably drifts back to those kitschy, animal-shaped terra-cotta figurines from the 1980s—chia seeds planted on the surface quickly sprout and resemble fur. Welcome to the chia of the 2000s, a new life for an old favorite. Although primarily grown in Mexico and Bolivia, chia seeds are rich in antioxidants, protein, and fiber, as well as omega-3 fatty acids. When exposed to liquid, the seeds turn gelatinous and develop a smooth coating. Gaining popularity to rival even that of flaxseed, chia has become the buzzy ingredient of the health food industry. Mixed in with fruits and vegetables and a little milk, the chia seed donates its burst of nutrition without altering the drink's full flavor because its flavor is neutral.

SERVINGS: 2
SERVING SIZE: 12 OZ

2 green Bartlett pears, peeled, cored, and sliced
1 cup unsweetened almond milk (or substitute unsweetened soy or coconut milk)
½ cup tightly packed baby spinach, stems removed
½ cup avocado, peeled, pitted, and chopped
1 teaspoon raw organic honey
1 teaspoon chia seeds
Juice of ½ small lime

Combine all ingredients in a blender and purée until smooth. Savor the flavor!

NUTRITIONAL INFORMATION PER SERVING: 181 cal., 5 g fat, 0 g sat. fat, 37 g carb., 3 g protein, 85 mg sodium, 22 g sugar, 8 g fiber.

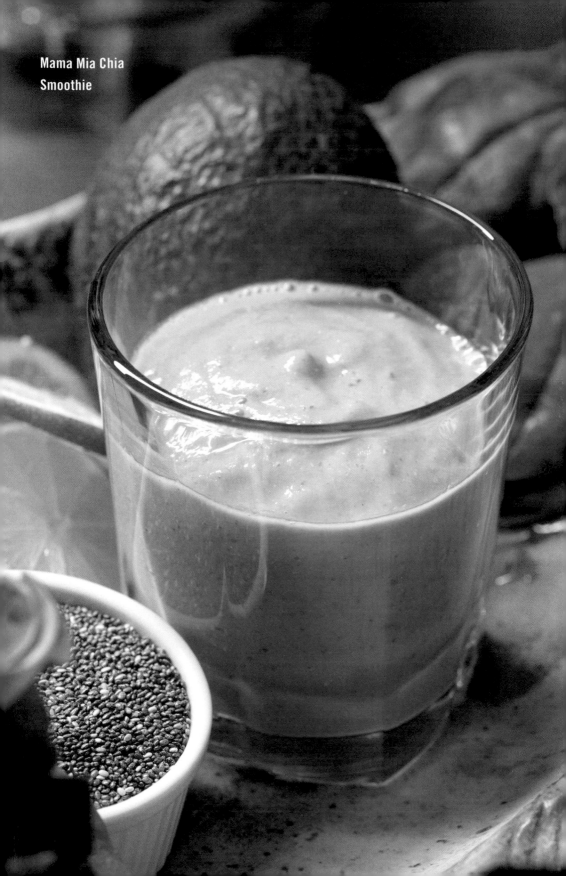

Mama Mia Chia
Smoothie

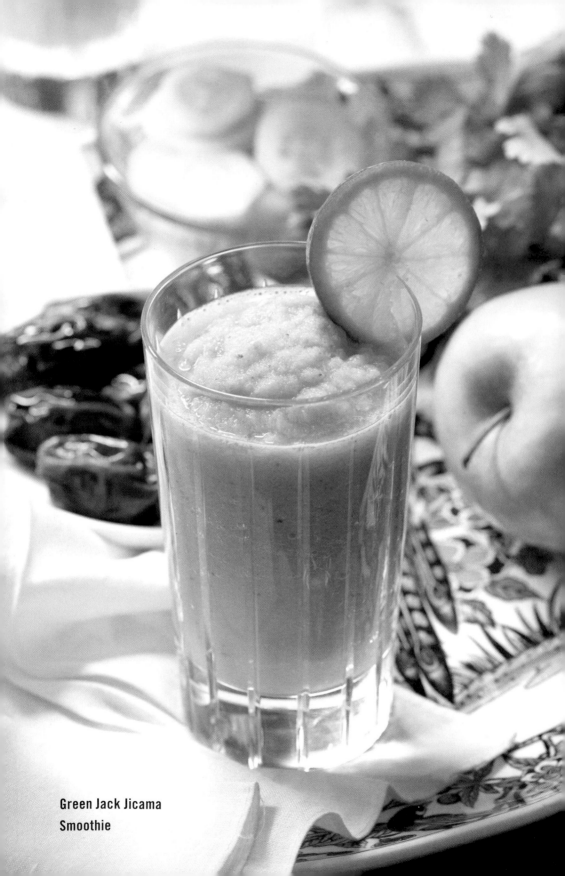

Green Jack Jicama
Smoothie

GREEN JACK JICAMA SMOOTHIE

No one would ever make the mistake of calling a jicama gorgeous. Often called the *Mexican water chestnut* or *yam bean*, its thick, tough skin is not only unappetizing but inedible. Washed just like potatoes, peeled, then cut into slices or chunks, jicama is versatile, low in calories, and high in nutrients. A powerhouse in its own right, jicama, with the crispness of an apple and a full, bright flavor, can jack up the heart-healthy potassium and vitamin C, as well as B vitamins such as riboflavin, thiamin, pyridoxine, and pantothenic acid.

SERVINGS: 2
SERVING SIZE: 12 OZ

1 cup cold-pressed apple juice (substitute fresh if available)
1 Granny Smith apple, peeled, cored, and sliced
½ cup peeled and chopped jicama
½ cup loosely packed curly kale, stems removed

One 6-inch piece cucumber, peeled and sliced, seeds can be left intact or removed
2 fresh pitted dates
Juice of 1 small lime
1 tablespoon chopped fresh cilantro leaves
10 small ice cubes

Combine all ingredients in a blender and purée until smooth. Delight in the rich taste!

NUTRITIONAL INFORMATION PER SERVING: 216 cal., 0 g fat, 0 g sat. fat, 54 g carb., 2 g protein, 14 mg sodium, 25 g sugar, 8 g fiber.

MEAN GREEN PROTEIN

Who doesn't like a good ole fashioned milkshake? The Mean Green Protein Shake takes what you love about the traditional and kicks it up to a modern level. No longer are shakes just about calories and sweetened saturated fats, the new shakes give you all kinds of health benefits and *still* taste great. This drink is full of protein and fiber, a great post workout drink or one to have any time during the day. Simple to make, easy on the palate, you will find this to be one of your go-to drinks when trying to fill the hunger void on a busy day.

SERVINGS: 2
SERVING SIZE: 12 OZ

2 Gala apples, peeled, cored, and sliced
1 ripe medium banana, peeled and sliced
½ cup chilled vanilla almond milk (or substitute unsweetened soy or coconut)

½ cup packed curly kale, stems removed
½ cup green seedless grapes
1 tablespoon organic vanilla hemp protein powder (or substitute with organic whey or pea protein powder)
¼ teaspoon ground cinnamon

Combine all ingredients with 1½ cup ice in a blender, and purée until smooth. Enjoy tremendously!

NUTRITIONAL INFORMATION PER SERVING: 218 cal., 1 g fat, 0 g sat. fat, 53 g carb., 4 g protein, 48 mg sodium, 35 g sugar, 8 g fiber.

GREEN TROPICAL TWISTER SMOOTHIE

This green smoothie comes with a refreshing tropical twist. Mango, pineapple, and banana flavors blend well with the kale to give a distinctively rich flavor. The mint is just enough to give it that island kick, conjuring images of oceanside relaxation with crystal-blue water just a few feet away. The frozen pineapples let a little sweetness linger in the aftertaste—and the coconut milk, with its iron, potassium, vitamin B3, and medium chain fatty acids, can help with everything from nerve communication to reducing insulin hormone resistance, a precursor to diabetes. This drink will have you smiling to the refrain, "Don't worry, be happy."

SERVINGS: 2
SERVING SIZE: 12 OZ

1 cup frozen pineapple chunks	½ cup tightly packed Lacinato
1 cup fresh or frozen peeled mango	(dinosaur) kale, stems removed
slices	½ ripe large banana, peeled and
¾ cup unsweetened almond milk (or	sliced
substitute unsweetened soy or	½ teaspoon chopped fresh mint
coconut milk)	leaves

Combine all ingredients in a blender and purée until smooth. Have fun!

NUTRITIONAL INFORMATION PER SERVING: 209 cal., 1 g fat, 0 g sat. fat, 51 g carb., 3 g protein, 61 mg sodium, 31 g sugar, 6 g fiber.

HER GREEN MAJESTY SMOOTHIE

Kale is one of the most potent healthy greens in the market. Full of vitamins A, C, and K and a nice dose of fiber, it's an ideal anchor when creating a healthy smoothie. Its slightly bitter, earthy taste is due to its high iron and can be nicely balanced with the sweetness of a banana and apple juice. Ginger also gets into the game to add spicy, pungent flavor. This strange-looking underground rhizome carries its own health punch, helping relieve gastrointestinal distress, lending strong antiinflammatory effects, and boosting the body's immune response. Kale may be the queen in this delicious smoothie, but her loyal court of nutrients is also to be admired.

SERVINGS: 2
SERVING SIZE: 12 OZ

1 ½ cups cold-pressed apple juice (substitute fresh if available)
1 cup loosely packed curly kale, stems removed
1 Bartlett pear, peeled, cored, and sliced
1 ripe small banana, peeled and sliced
½ cup avocado, peeled, pitted and chopped
One 5-inch piece cucumber, peeled and sliced, seeds can be left intact or removed
Juice of 1 large lemon
1 teaspoon peeled and grated ginger

Combine all ingredients in a blender and purée until smooth. Relish the rich flavors!

NUTRITIONAL INFORMATION PER SERVING: 295 cal., 6 g fat, 1 g sat. fat, 62 g carb., 4 g protein, 29 mg sodium, 40 g sugar, 9 g fiber.

GREEN SWIZZLE DETOX SMOOTHIE

Who says green drinks can't be fun and tasty? This smoothie is not your garden variety greenie. Yes, it delivers the fiber and other cleansing elements, but it also introduces ginger and lime to add to its flavor. Protein, calcium, and iron are the headlining nutrients in this drink. Dandelion greens add a nice twist to this smoothie. Not only are they loaded with antioxidants such as beta-carotene, but they also kick in copper, manganese, phosphorous, potassium, and magnesium. While their leaves are naturally bitter, the fruit that's mixed in with this drink does a great job of making it easy on the taste buds.

SERVINGS: 2
SERVING SIZE: 12 OZ

¾ cup unsweetened almond milk (or substitute unsweetened soy or coconut milk)
¾ cup frozen pineapple chunks
1 cup loosely packed chopped dandelion greens, stems removed
1 orange, peeled, sliced into sections, and seeded

1 ripe medium banana, peeled and sliced
1½ tablespoons unfiltered organic flaxseed oil
1 tablespoon raw organic honey (optional—will temper the bitterness of dandelions)
Juice of ½ small lime
½ teaspoon peeled and grated ginger

Combine all ingredients in a blender and purée until smooth. Enjoy every ounce!

NUTRITIONAL INFORMATION PER SERVING: 295 cal., 15 g fat, 2 g sat. fat, 53 g carb., 3 g protein, 97 mg sodium, 30 g sugar, 6 g fiber.

GREEN MANGO DETOX SMOOTHIE

Sometimes called the king of fruits, the mango with its bevy of nutritional elements is considered a super fruit. Exotic and tasty, the mango's sweetness with a prickle of tartness gives it a pleasant and rich flavor. The spinach in this drink will load you up with fiber, vitamins A, C, and K—and the mango, also rich in A and C, kicks in potassium, vitamin B6, and vitamin E. The pineapple give it a little sweetness, and the avocado provides a rich creamy texture. The blend of these distinct flavors makes detoxing fun and addictive.

SERVINGS: 2
SERVING SIZE: 12 OZ

1 cup chilled unsweetened coconut water
1 cup frozen pineapple chunks
1 cup fresh or frozen peeled mango slices
1 cup tightly packed spinach, stems removed
1 Gala apple, peeled, cored and sliced

1 small avocado, peeled, pitted, and chopped
1 teaspoon chopped fresh cilantro leaves
Juice of ½ small lemon
½ teaspoon peeled and grated ginger

Combine all ingredients in a blender and purée until smooth. Enjoy!

NUTRITIONAL INFORMATION PER SERVING: 263 cal., 7 g fat, 1 g sat. fat, 51 g carb., 3 g protein, 78 mg sodium, 30 g sugar, 9 g fiber.

THE ALKALINE GODDESS

Our bodies are in a constant tug of war between acidity and alkalinity. Usually you are in an alkaline state with your body's pH typically registering somewhere between 7.35 and 7.40. Too much acid prompts your body to find a balance, and this means draining your bones of nutrients. Leafy greens, cucumbers, avocados, and limes are just some of the many alkaline foods that we can eat to keep pH in the zone that our bodies crave for optimal health. The Alkaline Goddess not only exerts its nutritional prowess, but she brings earthly pleasure to your taste buds as well.

SERVINGS: 2
SERVING SIZE: 12 OZ

1 cup chilled unsweetened coconut water

1 cup frozen blueberries

½ cup cold-pressed apple juice (substitute fresh if available)

1 small avocado, peeled, pitted, and chopped

1 ripe small banana, peeled and sliced

One 4-inch piece cucumber, peeled and sliced (optional to remove or leave seeds)

½ cup tightly packed curly kale, stems removed

Juice of 1 small lime

2 teaspoons organic vanilla hemp protein powder (organic whey or pea protein optional)

Combine all ingredients in a blender and purée until smooth. Relish the luscious flavors!

NUTRITIONAL INFORMATION PER SERVING: 258 cal., 8 g fat, 1 g sat. fat, 44 g carb., 6 g protein, 111 mg sodium, 27 g sugar, 10 g fiber.

APPLE ZAPPER SMOOTHIE

Apples can make almost any smoothie taste delicious, but Honeycrisp apples, first developed back in the 1930s at the University of Minnesota, possibly the most. Universally enjoyed for its sweetness, the apple's relatively neutral taste allows it to be a great companion to other flavors when combined in a drink. Carrots deliver a generous supply of vitamin A, vitamin B6, vitamin K, fiber, vitamin C, and potassium. Throw in a little ginger to soothe your gastrointestinal tract and stimulate digestion, circulation, and sweating. All of these ingredients combined make a potent and tasty health elixir.

SERVINGS: 2
SERVING SIZE: 12 OZ

2 large Honeycrisp apples, peeled, cored, and quartered
1 cup chilled unsweetened coconut water
½ cup cold-pressed apple juice (substitute fresh if available)
½ cup tightly packed curly kale, stems removed
½ small lime, peeled, sliced into sections, and seeded
½ small carrot, peeled and sliced
1 tablespoon unfiltered organic flaxseed oil
⅛ teaspoon peeled and grated ginger
8 small ice cubes

Combine the ingredients in a blender and purée until smooth. Smile as you drink!

NUTRITIONAL INFORMATION PER SERVING: 238 cal., 7 g fat, 1 g sat. fat, 46 g carb., 1 g protein, 71 mg sodium, 34 g sugar, 6 g fiber.

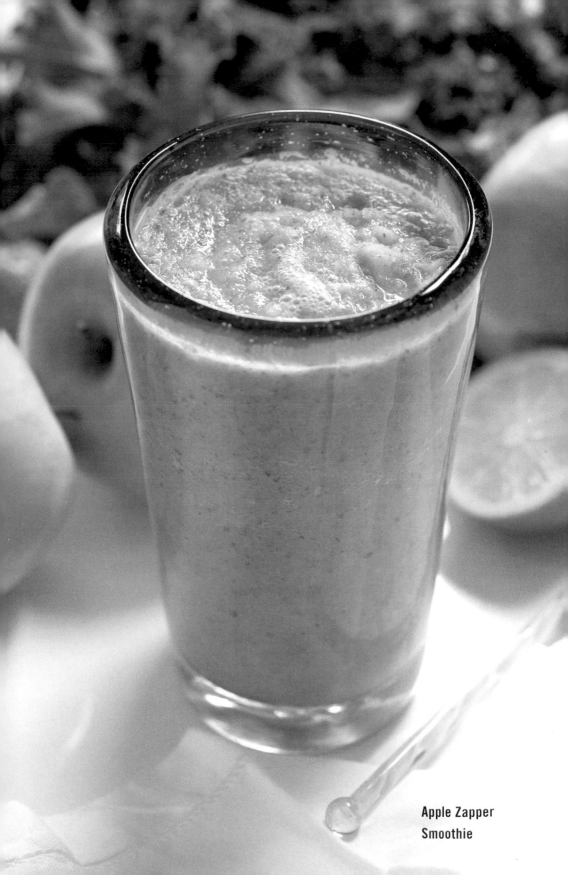

Apple Zapper
Smoothie

SWEET-AND-SOUR DETOX SMOOTHIE

Get the best of both worlds: Sweet *and* Sour pack a great detox punch! The natural sweetness of bananas and oranges balance the sour flavor of lemons and limes. Citrus fruits have been touted for their cleansing properties, but adding spinach to the mix makes this drink an even more powerful detox. The busy little enzymes in this drink will activate enzymes in the liver to boost its already important cleansing properties. The fiber can help scrub the intestines, which also are one of the most important organs in the body's natural detoxifying process. Chock full of vitamins and minerals such as vitamins B, K, and E—as well as manganese, copper, magnesium, and phosphorous—just one drink will send your body into healthy overdrive.

SERVINGS: 2
SERVING SIZE: 12 OZ

1 cup loosely packed baby spinach, stems removed	½ small lemon, peeled, sliced into sections, and seeded
1 ripe medium banana, peeled and sliced	½ small lime, peeled, sliced into sections, and seeded
½ cup low-fat plain yogurt	2 tablespoons unfiltered organic flaxseed oil
½ cup fresh orange juice	

Combine all ingredients in a blender with 8 ice cubes and purée until smooth. Drink and have fun!

NUTRITIONAL INFORMATION PER SERVING: 248 cal., 15 g fat, 2 g sat. fat, 27 g carb., 5 g protein, 56 mg sodium, 17 g sugar, 2 g fiber.

GREEN MANIA SMOOTHIE

Green is the color of health. Full of fiber and vitamins K, A, and C, this three-greens drink is truly the mother lode of health. There's also protein, iron, calcium, and magnesium to round out the smorgasbord of nutrients that make this smoothie a true pillar of the cleanse. Apples and pears bring up the fiber count and the sweetness as well, adding very little in the way of calories but lots in the way of flavor and powerful phytonutrients.

SERVINGS: 2
SERVING SIZE: 12 OZ

2 Bosc pears, peeled, cored, and sliced

2 medium Granny Smith apples, peeled, cored, and sliced

1 cup unsweetened almond milk (or substitute unsweetened soy or coconut milk)

1 cup frozen pineapple chunks

½ cup tightly packed curly kale, stems removed

½ cup packed baby spinach, stems removed

1 teaspoon fresh mint leaves

Combine the ingredients in a blender with 8 ice cubes and purée until smooth. Relish the flavors!

NUTRITIONAL INFORMATION PER SERVING: 221 cal., 2 g fat, 0 g sat. fat, 54 g carb., 3 g protein, 13 mg sodium, 37 g sugar, 8 g fiber.

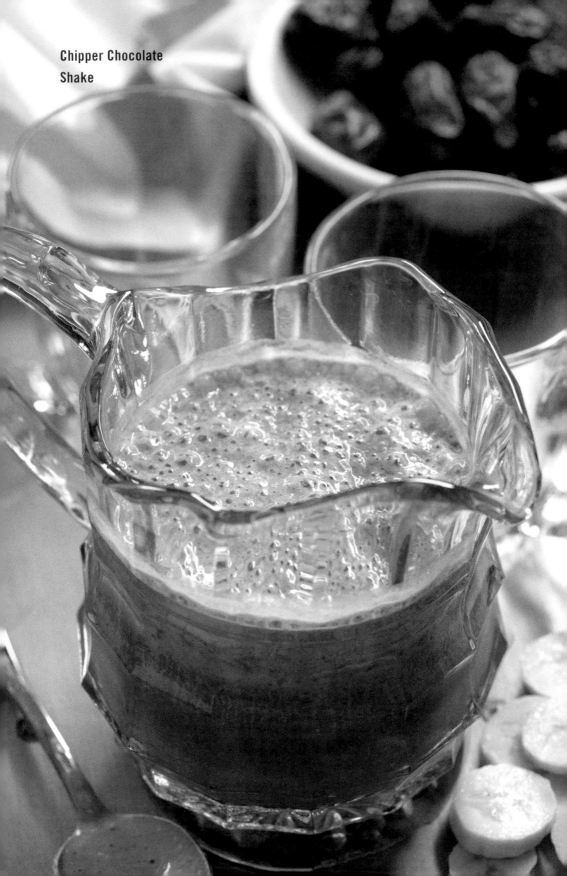

Chipper Chocolate
Shake

CHIPPER CHOCOLATE SHAKE

The chocolate milk shake is an iconic drink for chocolate lovers everywhere. But that rich, creamy flavor comes at great calorie cost. This lower calorie version takes out the ice cream but keeps the flavor and thickness. The dates provide a little fiber and sweetness. The ingredient list is simple and delicious. There's nothing like filling up on half the calories and satisfying your taste buds at the same time.

SERVINGS: 2
SERVING SIZE: 12 OZ

1½ cups 2 percent reduced-fat chocolate milk
1 ripe small banana, peeled and sliced
1½ pitted dates

2 tablespoons nonfat chocolate yogurt
1 tablespoon sweetened cocoa powder (or 2 tablespoons for a stronger chocolate flavor)
12 small ice cubes

Combine all ingredients in a blender and purée until smooth. Enjoy and be happy!

NUTRITIONAL INFORMATION PER SERVING: 241 cal., 4 g fat, 2 g sat. fat, 47 g carb., 8 g protein, 194 mg sodium, 26 g sugar, 4 g fiber.

PURPLE STINGER SMOOTHIE

What's not to like about this drink? Sweet, filling, tasty, and so easy to make. Drink it fresh or take it on the go. Loaded with fiber and with the secret added ingredient of fresh bee pollen, Purple Stinger Smoothie not only will enhance your body's natural cleansing abilities but can also help prime the soldiers of your immune system to fight off potential disease-causing invaders. This eclectic combination of ingredients provides a smooth drink that will leave you satisfied and energized.

SERVINGS: 2
SERVING SIZE: 12 OZ

1 cup unsweetened almond milk (or substitute unsweetened soy or coconut milk)
1 cup frozen blueberries
1 cup sliced fresh strawberries (substitute frozen if fresh are not available)
1 cup tightly packed chopped Swiss chard, stems removed

1 ripe small banana, peeled and sliced
One 3-inch piece cucumber, peeled and sliced
Juice of ½ large lemon
½ teaspoon organic bee pollen granules

Combine the ingredients in a blender and purée until smooth. Feel energized!

NUTRITIONAL INFORMATION PER SERVING: 153 cal., 2 g fat, 0 g sat. fat, 34 g carb., 3 g protein, 116 mg sodium, 21 g sugar, 6 g fiber.

RECIPE NOTE: Bee pollen is one of nature's most nourishing foods, with approximately 40% of its composition being protein, greater than any other animal source. It also contains free amino acids and vitamins, including the B-complex and folic acid. Scientists consider bee pollen to be a complete food, full of all the essential elements for life. Make sure you choose organic bee pollen and get it from a reputable health food store to make sure it is of high quality.

MIGHTY FEROCIOUS FIBER SMOOTHIE

Beans are a great source of protein and fiber. They give you energy and they make you feel full on fewer calories. Mixing them with fruit gives a unique taste and texture that is extremely healthy and refreshing at the same time. Chia seeds, with their mild, nutty flavor, are a whole grain, adding fiber and protein to make this a powerful drink. The real bonus with this drink is that you can consume as much as a third of your day's recommended amount of fiber in 1 serving.

SERVINGS: 2
SERVING SIZE: 12 OZ

1½ cups frozen pineapple chunks
1 cup tightly packed kale,
    stems removed
¾ cup unsweetened almond milk
    (or substitute unsweetened soy
    or coconut milk)
1 ripe banana, peeled, sliced,
    and frozen

½ cup canned cannellini beans,
    rinsed and drained
½ cup frozen raspberries
2 tablespoons nonfat
    strawberry yogurt
1 teaspoon chia seeds

Combine all ingredients in a blender and purée until smooth. Drink and be energized!

NUTRITIONAL INFORMATION PER SERVING: 258 cal., 3 g fat, 0 g sat. fat, 54 g carb., 8 g protein, 96 mg sodium, 16 g sugar, 9 g fiber.

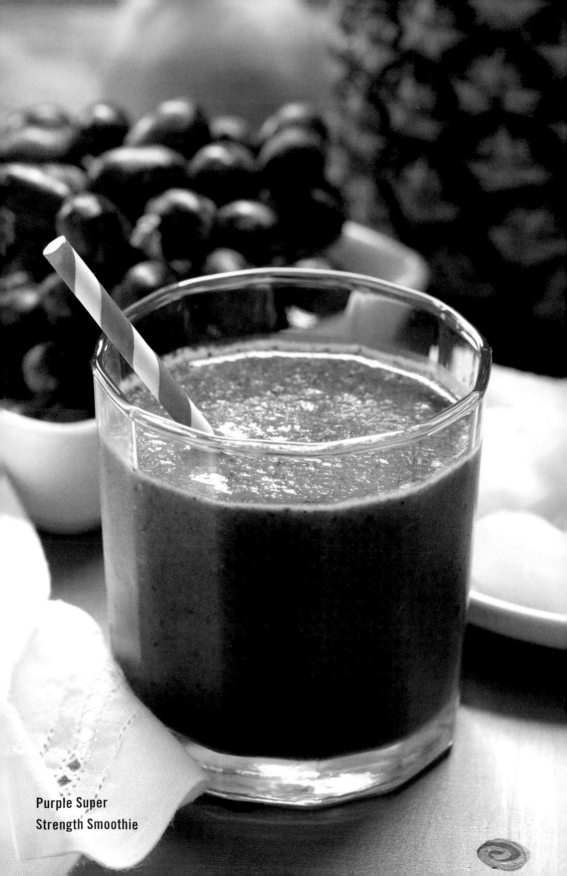

Purple Super
Strength Smoothie

PURPLE SUPER STRENGTH SMOOTHIE

The power of purple is evident in this delightfully sweet drink that combines many strange bedfellows. Black grapes, a pear, pineapple chunks, and baby spinach are an unusual but killer combination. Throw them all in a blender with a little flaxseed oil, and you have a purple detox smoothie that keeps the calorie count down while raising the roof on the antioxidant levels. Full of super foods and supreme taste, you'll start feeling good after the first sip.

SERVINGS: 2
SERVING SIZE: 12 OZ

1½ cups cold-pressed apple juice (substitute fresh if available)
1 cup black seedless grapes
1 Bartlett pear, peeled, cored, and sliced
½ cup frozen pineapple chunks
½ cup tightly packed baby spinach, stems removed
1 tablespoon unfiltered organic flaxseed oil

Combine all ingredients in a blender and purée until smooth. Enjoy your creation!

NUTRITIONAL INFORMATION PER SERVING: 228 cal., 7 g fat, 1 g sat. fat, 43 g carb., 1 g protein, 11 mg sodium, 30 g sugar, 5 g fiber.

MIDNIGHT MADNESS SMOOTHIE

The dark color of this smoothie is a testament to the richness of the flavor, as well as the wealth of health benefits it offers. Who knew that black beans could be as tasty in a smoothie as they could be in a bowl of hot soup? And the powers of black beans are legendary—almost 15 grams of fiber and 15 grams of protein in 1 cup! Combine this with the antioxidant properties of berries, and this is a drink that not only keeps you full for a long time but increases your energy and ability to fight disease. The hemp seeds contain all of the essential amino acids, making them ideal as a vegetarian protein. Iron, potassium, vitamin E, magnesium, and fiber are also contained in this tiny seed and add power to this drink.

SERVINGS: 2
SERVING SIZE: 12 OZ

1 cup mixed 100% berry juice (combination of berries that could include: blueberry, blackberry, strawberry, cranberry or raspberry)
1 cup frozen blueberries
1 cup tightly packed baby spinach, stems removed
1 frozen banana, peeled and sliced
¾ cup frozen pitted cherries
½ cup canned black beans, rinsed and drained
1 teaspoon organic vanilla hemp protein powder (or substitute organic whey or pea protein powder)
6 small ice cubes

Combine all ingredients in a blender and purée until smooth. Enjoy!

NUTRITIONAL INFORMATION PER SERVING: 235 cal., 1 g fat, 0 g sat. fat, 53 g carb., 6 g protein, 28 mg sodium, 32 g sugar, 8 g fiber.

UTOPIA SMOOTHIE

There's nothing like detoxing amid a wash of natural sweetness. The Utopia Smoothie is the answer for those who don't want to feel like they're eating grass when trying to boost their body's natural cleansing ability. Yes, it's possible to have a healthy drink that also tastes sweet and rich. This smoothie delivers as much as a third of your recommended daily intake of fiber, and acts like a scrub brush on your intestinal tract, steadily cleansing throughout its journey. Make sure you mince your ginger as finely as possible so that the spice physically gets lost in the smoothie, but its taste happily lingers.

SERVINGS: 2
SERVING SIZE: 12 OZ

1½ cups Bartlett pears, peeled, cored, and sliced (other types can be used if preferred)
1 cup frozen strawberries (substitute fresh if desired)
¾ cup frozen blueberries
½ cup cold-pressed apple juice (substitute fresh if available)

2 tablespoons low-fat strawberry yogurt
1 tablespoon unfiltered organic flaxseed oil
⅛ teaspoon peeled and grated ginger

Combine the ingredients in a blender and purée until smooth. Drink enthusiastically!

NUTRITIONAL INFORMATION PER SERVING: 230 cal., 7 g fat, 1 g sat. fat, 44 g carb., 2 g protein, 14 mg sodium, 29 g sugar, 8 g fiber.

WHOLE-GRAIN EXTRAVAGANZA SMOOTHIE

There's nothing more filling than a serving of whole grains, full of all types of nutrients including protein, fiber, iron, magnesium, copper, and manganese. Containing all three essential parts of the kernel—bran, germ, and endosperm—oats rank in the top echelon of whole grains. A leader in calcium, manganese, fiber, and protein, oats deliver a tremendous nutritional value without loading on the calories. As if the concoction couldn't get any healthier, throw in a little flaxseed for heart-healthy omega-3 fatty acids, then sprinkle in some macadamia nuts for their sweet taste, rich fiber, and mono-unsaturated fatty acids that lowers the bad cholesterol (LDL) and increases the good cholesterol (HDL).

SERVINGS: 2
SERVING SIZE: 12 OZ

1¼ cups unsweetened almond milk (or substitute unsweetened soy or coconut milk)
1 Gala apple, peeled, cored, and sliced
1 ripe banana, peeled, sliced, and frozen

¾ cup old-fashioned rolled oats
4 tablespoons nonfat vanilla yogurt
1 tablespoon unfiltered organic flaxseed oil
6 small ice cubes

Combine all ingredients in a blender and purée until smooth. Enjoy!

NUTRITIONAL INFORMATION PER SERVING: 295 cal., 11 g fat, 1 g sat. fat, 52 g carb., 6 g protein, 120 mg sodium, 22 g sugar, 6 g fiber.

CHOCOLATE BLUEBERRY SMOOTHIE

No, you haven't misread anything. Two of our tastiest treats can be enjoyed on the SHRED Power Cleanse. You think chocolate-covered strawberries are good? Wait until you taste the combo of chocolate and blueberries. There's no better way to satisfy your sweet tooth, as well as load up on antioxidants, fiber, and some protein for good measure. Throw in some white beans to pump up the fiber and protein, and you have what many would consider an almost perfect health-boosting smoothie. This eclectic array of ingredients may sound like strange bedfellows, but when combined they bring out the best in each other.

SERVINGS: 2
SERVING SIZE: 12 OZ

1 cup frozen blueberries
1 cup unsweetened almond milk (or substitute unsweetened soy or coconut milk)
1 ripe small banana, peeled and sliced
½ cup tightly packed curly kale, stems removed
2 tablespoons cup unsweetened dark chocolate chips
2 tablespoons nonfat blueberry yogurt
¼ cup cooked low-sodium white beans
1 tablespoon sweetened ground baking cocoa powder
1 teaspoon raw organic honey
¼ teaspoon pure vanilla extract

Combine all ingredients in a blender and purée until smooth. Drink and savor the taste!

NUTRITIONAL INFORMATION PER SERVING: 298 cal., 14 g fat, 10 g sat. fat, 38 g carb., 7 g protein, 104 mg sodium, 20 g sugar, 9 g fiber.

SWEET DETOX SMOOTHIE

If you like sweet, you'll love this drink. A gorgeous concoction of berries and pears mixed with fresh juice and some ice to thicken everything up. The sweetness comes from the natural sugars that are found in the berries and pears; the flaxseed oil provides a healthy dose of disease-preventing omega-3 fatty acids, and yogurt kicks in calcium. From the dark rich-purple color to the refreshing sweetness to the energizing nutrients, there's nothing not to like in this simple blend.

SERVINGS: 2
SERVING SIZE: 12 OZ

1 cup cold-pressed apple juice
   (substitute fresh if available,
   or use cold water to make
   the smoothie less sweet)
1 cup frozen blueberries
1 cup sliced Bosc or Bartlett pears,
   peeled, cored, and sliced

½ cup sliced fresh strawberries
   (substitute frozen if fresh
   are not available)
2 tablespoons nonfat strawberry
   yogurt
1 tablespoon unfiltered organic
   flaxseed oil
6 small ice cubes

Combine all ingredients in a blender and purée until smooth. Drink with a smile!

NUTRITIONAL INFORMATION PER SERVING: 219 cal., 8 g fat, 1 g sat. fat, 39 g carb., 1 g protein, 13 mg sodium, 27 g sugar, 5 g fiber.

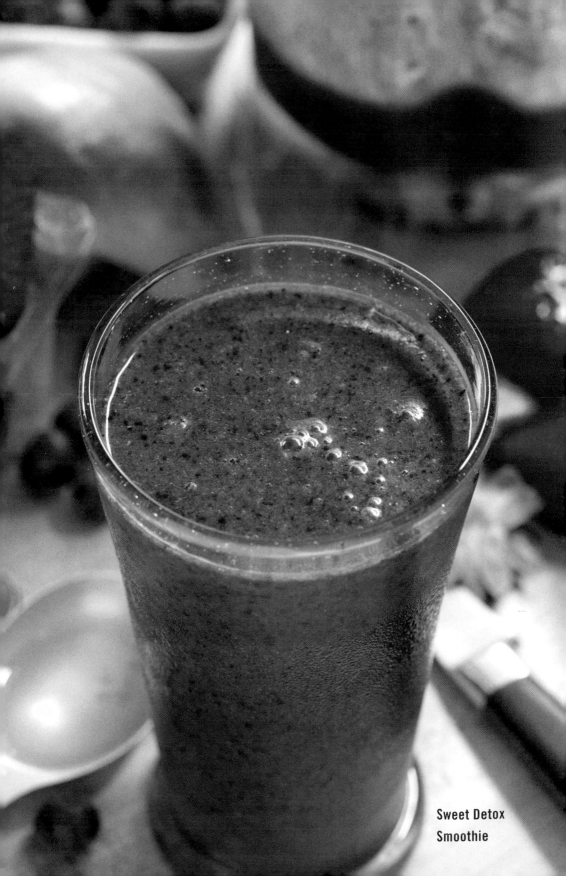

Sweet Detox
Smoothie

RASPBERRY CHIA SMOOTHIE

Chia is a flowering plant in the mint family native to Mexico and Guatemala. The seeds were an important food for the Aztecs. These little seeds are a dynamo of nutrition containing fiber, protein, calcium, manganese, phosphorous, and healthy omega-3 fats. The combination of chia seeds with raspberries not only bumps up the antioxidant quotient but also blends in a natural sweetness. The chickpeas really help boost the protein count, and you'll never notice them in this juicy red concoction.

SERVINGS: 2
SERVING SIZE: 12 OZ

1½ cup frozen strawberries (substitute fresh if desired)
½ cup cold-pressed apple juice (substitute fresh if available)
½ medium ripe banana, peeled and sliced
¼ cup canned chickpeas, rinsed and drained (optional)
¼ cup old-fashioned rolled oats
3 tablespoons low-fat or nonfat vanilla Greek yogurt
1 tablespoon chia seeds, soaked in water for 5 minutes
⅛ teaspoon ground cinnamon
10 small ice cubes

Combine all ingredients in a blender and purée until smooth. Enjoy!

NUTRITIONAL INFORMATION PER SERVING: 248 cal., 4 g fat, 1 g sat. fat, 47 g carb., 9 g protein, 22 mg sodium, 16 g sugar, 9 g fiber.

ALL-AROUND SMOOTHIE

Remember the kid in high school who seemed to play every sport with ease and finesse? This smoothie is that kid. From apples to mangoes to hemp hearts to bananas, this meal in a glass gives you the best of everything. Fiber, protein, omega-3 fatty acids, and a complement of vitamins: this is truly an all-star version of liquid health.

SERVINGS: 2
SERVING SIZE: 12 OZ

1 cup fresh orange juice
1 large Gala apple, peeled, cored, and sliced
½ cup tightly packed curly kale, stems removed
½ cup sliced fresh strawberries (substitute frozen if desired)
½ medium ripe banana, peeled and sliced
¼ cup fresh or frozen peeled mango slices
⅛ cup chopped celery stalks
1 teaspoon organic vanilla hemp protein powder (or substitute organic whey or pea protein powder)

Combine all ingredients in a blender and purée until smooth. Relish the great flavors!

NUTRITIONAL INFORMATION PER SERVING: 182 cal., 0 g fat, 0 g sat. fat, 45 g carb., 3 g protein, 14 mg sodium, 32 g sugar, 5 g fiber.

WORKOUT WARRIOR SMOOTHIE

Physical exertion requires energy in order to maximize the benefits of the activity. So it's not surprising that priming your pump before strenuous exercise is the smartest strategy before your workout. The same, however, is true *after* a workout. The type of fuel you replace after exertion is essential to the repair that occurs after exercise. This smoothie is truly ambidextrous in the sense that it can be used both pre- and post-workout. It's full of antioxidants, a barrage of vitamins and minerals that can help increase energy levels, and a protein punch to help build more of that lean muscle mass that keeps you burning calories even while resting. This smoothie will turn you into a workout warrior, and your body will have no choice but to respond.

SERVINGS: 2
SERVING SIZE: 12 OZ

1 cup frozen blueberries
1 cup strawberries (substitute frozen if fresh are not available)
½ cup unsweetened almond milk (or substitute unsweetened soy or coconut milk)
½ cup mixed 100% berry juice (combination of berries that could include: blueberry, blackberry, strawberry, cranberry or raspberry)

½ ripe medium banana, peeled and sliced
¼ cup low-fat or fat-free blueberry Greek yogurt
¼ cup fresh raspberries (substitute frozen if fresh are not available)
¼ cup old-fashioned rolled oats
1 tablespoon unfiltered organic flaxseed oil
½ teaspoon raw organic honey (optional, as a sweetener)

Combine all ingredients in a blender and purée until smooth. Enjoy!

NUTRITIONAL INFORMATION PER SERVING: 278 cal., 9 g fat, 1 g sat. fat, 47 g carb., 5 g protein, 55 mg sodium, 31 g sugar, 7 g fiber.

NO HASSLE SWEET SMOOTHIE

The combination of blueberries and pineapples can never be wrong. These two strong, distinct flavors work together to create a sweet mixture that is thickened and improved with strawberry yogurt. The apple juice gives the smoothie a sweet base, and the kale and flaxseed punch up the fiber quotient to make this drink appealing to the eye as well as the taste buds.

SERVINGS: 2
SERVING SIZE: 12 OZ

1 cup cold-pressed apple juice
  (substitute fresh if available)
1 cup frozen blueberries
1 cup frozen pineapple chunks
½ cup loosely packed Lacinato
  (dinosaur) kale, stems removed

2 tablespoons nonfat
  strawberry yogurt
1 tablespoon unfiltered organic
  flaxseed oil

Combine all ingredients in a blender and purée until smooth. Drink with satisfaction!

NUTRITIONAL INFORMATION PER SERVING: 221 cal., 8 g fat, 1 g sat. fat, 39 g carb., 2 g protein, 17 mg sodium, 23 g sugar, 5 g fiber.

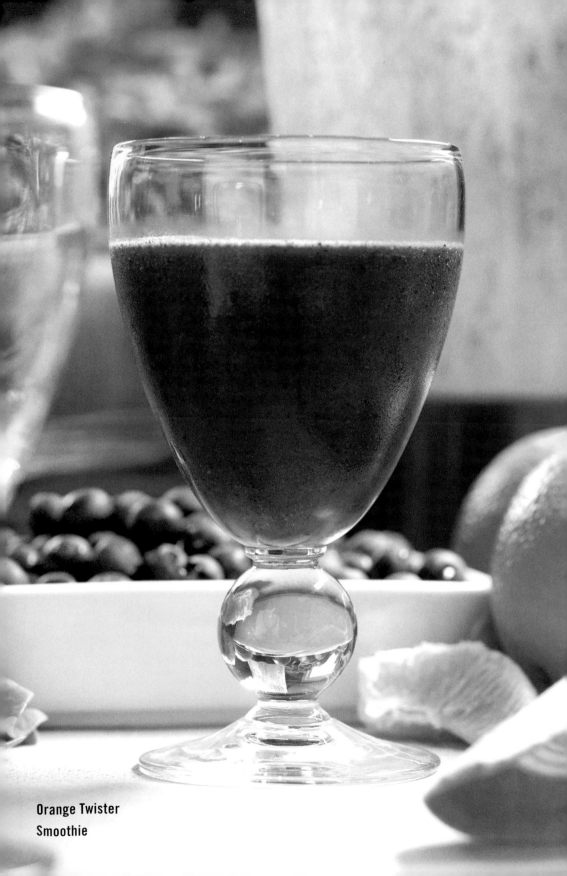

Orange Twister
Smoothie

ORANGE TWISTER SMOOTHIE

This medley of fibrous fruits is an antioxidant powerhouse. Loaded with vitamin C and respectable contributions of other nutrients such as magnesium and potassium, this drink enhances your body's physiology after seducing you with its sweet aroma and reddish-orange hue. For just 139 calories, you get 2 grams of protein and 3 grams of fiber and enough bulk to keep you full until the next meal.

SERVINGS: 2
SERVING SIZE: 12 OZ

½ cup fresh orange juice
Juice of 1 large Valencia orange (or
    substitute navel or juice orange)
½ cup frozen blueberries
½ cup frozen raspberries
½ cup frozen strawberry slices

½ cup tightly packed Swiss chard,
    stems removed
1 tablespoon unfiltered organic
    flaxseed oil
10 small ice cubes

Combine all ingredients in a blender and purée until smooth. Enjoy the experience!

NUTRITIONAL INFORMATION PER SERVING: 139 cal., 7 g fat, 1 g sat. fat, 19 g carb., 2 g protein, 20 mg sodium, 12 g sugar, 3 g fiber.

CHOCOLATE PARADISE SMOOTHIE

The thick rich flavor of chocolate has delighted people since 1900 BCE in Mesoamerica. The raw cacao seeds were so valuable that they were used as a form of currency. What was known in ancient times is confirmed by modern research. The cacao bean contains flavonoids, powerful antioxidants that can help neutralize and destroy free radicals that can cause cell injury and serious illness. Mix these antioxidants with the sweetness of dates and you now have a winning combo. Dates are serious health promoters in their own right, full of potassium, calcium, manganese, iron, fiber—and their own version of antioxidants, which are called *tannins*. Savor the flavor and enjoy the health wonders of this drink.

SERVINGS: 2
SERVING SIZE: 12 OZ

1 cup frozen strawberry slices
1 ripe medium banana, peeled, sliced, and frozen
½ cup fat-free chocolate milk

1½ pitted dates
2 tablespoons nonfat plain yogurt
1 tablespoon cocoa powder
10 small ice cubes

Combine all ingredients in a blender and purée until smooth. Drink with pleasure!

NUTRITIONAL INFORMATION PER SERVING: 177 cal., 1 g fat, 0 g sat. fat, 43 g carb., 4 g protein, 65 mg sodium, 18 g sugar, 6 g fiber.

THE BLUEBERRY TORNADO

Ranked second only to strawberries as the most popular berry in the US, blueberries are a heavyweight fighter when it comes to antioxidant capacity. Raw, uncooked blueberries provide not only the best flavor but also the greatest number of nutritional benefits. Along with the ability to wage war against the dangerous free radicals, a cup of blueberries provides a significant amount of vitamin K, vitamin C, manganese, and fiber. This smoothie bumps up the nutritional power with hemp protein powder and flaxseed oil, their nutty flavors swallowed up by the swirling sweetness of the blueberries and banana.

SERVINGS: 2
SERVING SIZE: 12 OZ

1 cup chilled coconut water (substitute cold-pressed apple juice if you prefer a sweeter drink)
1 cup fresh blueberries (substitute frozen if fresh are not available)
1 ripe small banana, peeled and sliced
½ cup loosely packed spinach, stems removed
Juice of 1 small lemon
2 tablespoons unfiltered organic flaxseed oil
10 small ice cubes

Combine the ingredients in a blender and purée until smooth. Luxuriate in the flavors!

NUTRITIONAL INFORMATION PER SERVING: 238 cal., 14 g fat, 2 g sat. fat, 30 g carb., 2 g protein, 67 mg sodium, 19 g sugar, 4 g fiber.

THE TRANQUILIZER

This drink is all about soothing. Kefir is a nutritious dairy product that is enzyme-rich and filled with probiotics, micro-organisms friendly with your gut's "inner ecosystem." More nutritious than its cousin yogurt, kefir also provides complete protein, important minerals, and a host of critical B vitamins. And it tastes tart and refreshing. Pineapple and peaches throw in fiber, as well as a natural sweetness that makes the drink as tasty as it is healthy. Even those who are lactose-intolerant might find this drink enjoyable; the kefir contains lactase, an enzyme that consumes most of the remaining lactose.

SERVINGS: 2
SERVING SIZE: 12 OZ

1 cup peeled, seeded, and chopped papaya	½ cup unsweetened coconut milk (or substitute unsweetened almond or soy milk)
½ cup frozen pineapple chunks (substitute fresh if desired)	Juice of ½ small lime
½ cup frozen peach slices (substitute fresh if desired)	1 tablespoon unfiltered organic flaxseed oil
½ cup low-fat plain kefir	½ tablespoon raw organic honey

Combine all ingredients in a blender and purée until smooth. Enjoy!

NUTRITIONAL INFORMATION PER SERVING: 270 cal., 18 g fat, 10 g sat. fat, 28 g carb., 4 g protein, 59 mg sodium, 16 g sugar, 3 g fiber.

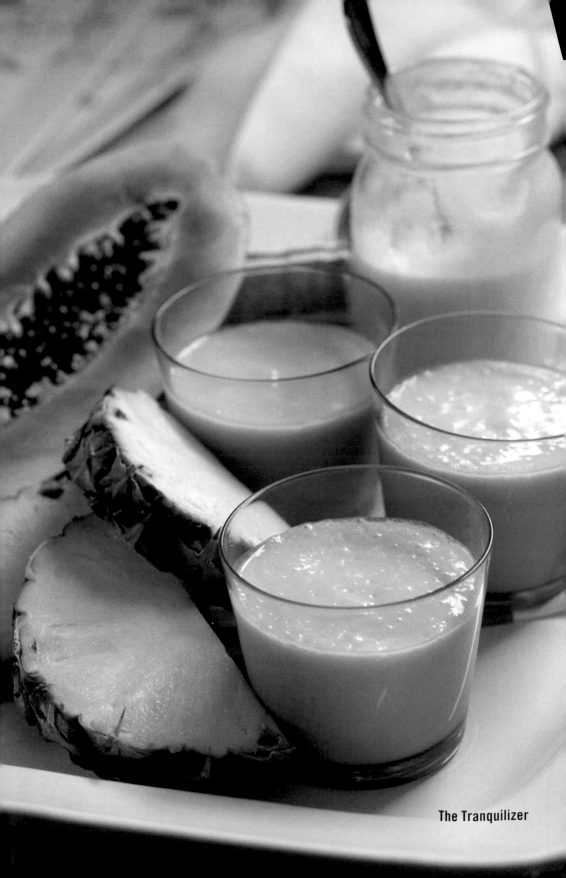

The Tranquilizer

CHOCOLATE RAZZY SMOOTHIE

This smoothie features a dream combination of chocolate and raspberries. Even better, the heavy dose of protein and the healthy fiber load make it great for your body. The raspberries deliver both fiber and sweetness. The chia seeds donate fiber and powerful omega-3 fatty acids. The banana does its job of kicking in fiber too, as well as a host of vitamins like C and B6 on top of potassium. This drink is a healthy way to answer a craving for chocolate. If you want to make this smoothie even thicker, soak the chia seeds in water for an hour. If you want them more plump, soak them overnight, and then add them with the other ingredients.

SERVINGS: 2
SERVING SIZE: 12 OZ

1 cup unsweetened coconut milk (or substitute unsweetened almond or soy milk)
1 cup frozen raspberries
1 small ripe banana, peeled and sliced
¼ cup chilled water
2 tablespoons low-fat or fat-free raspberry yogurt

1 tablespoon semisweet dark chocolate chips
2 teaspoons unfiltered organic flaxseed oil
1½ teaspoons organic chocolate hemp protein powder (or substitute organic chocolate whey protein powder)
1 teaspoon ground chia seeds
10 small ice cubes

Combine all ingredients in a blender and purée until smooth. Drink your creation with pleasure!

NUTRITIONAL INFORMATION PER SERVING: 167 cal., 11 g fat, 8 g sat. fat, 29 g carb., 3 g protein, 44 mg sodium, 15 g sugar, 7 g fiber.

ENERGETIC KALACIOUS SMOOTHIE

Many think that cleansing means the loss of energy. But nothing can be further from the truth when you load up on the right ingredients. Kale, one of the healthiest leafy greens, never lets you down. Its taste can be a little earthy for some, but mixing it with sweet peaches and berries can liven up its flavor and remind you how healthy it is with all of its vitamin A, C, and K. Flaxseed slides quietly into this drink, but loudly delivers fiber, vitamin B1, copper, and omega-3 fatty acids. The lemon generously throws in a heaping amount of vitamin C and folate, giving this smoothie an extra little zip.

SERVINGS: 2
SERVING SIZE: 12 OZ

1 cup frozen mixed berries (such as raspberries, strawberries, cherries, and blackberries)	1 small kiwi, peeled and sliced
	½ cup tightly packed Swiss chard, stems removed
1 cup tightly packed curly or Lacinato (dinosaur) kale, stems removed	¼ cup chopped celery stalks
	Juice of ½ small lemon
½ cup cold-pressed apple juice (substitute fresh if available)	2 tablespoons unfiltered organic flaxseed oil
½ cup frozen peach slices (or substitute fresh peaches if desired)	1 teaspoon organic vanilla hemp protein powder (or substitute with organic whey or pea protein powder)
1 ripe small banana, peeled and sliced	

Combine all ingredients in a blender and purée until smooth. Drink with pleasure!

NUTRITIONAL INFORMATION PER SERVING: 296 cal., 14 g fat, 2 g sat. fat, 42 g carb., 3 g protein, 29 mg sodium, 25 g sugar, 6 g fiber.

THE GREEN GRAPE-ANATOR

This is a revitalizing smoothie. The lime juice not only helps the liver in its cleansing duties, but its high amount of vitamin C prompts the liver to make glutathione, one of the most powerful of the antioxidants. Cilantro pulls its fair share of the cleansing work by binding toxic metals in a process called *chelation*. The Green Grape-anator doesn't just help your body detox, but it also loads you up with an assortment of phytonutrients that will deliver a boost of energy.

SERVINGS: 2
SERVING SIZE: 12 OZ

2 cups green seedless grapes, frozen	½ ripe small banana, peeled and sliced
½ cup cold-pressed apple juice (substitute fresh if available)	Juice of ½ small lime
	2 tablespoons nonfat plain yogurt
½ cup tightly packed Swiss chard, stems removed	1 teaspoon chopped fresh cilantro leaves
	10 small ice cubes

Combine the ingredients in a blender and purée until smooth. Drink and bask in the flavors!

NUTRITIONAL INFORMATION PER SERVING: 187 cal., 0 g fat, 0 g sat. fat, 48 g carb., 3 g protein, 28 mg sodium, 36 g sugar, 3 g fiber.

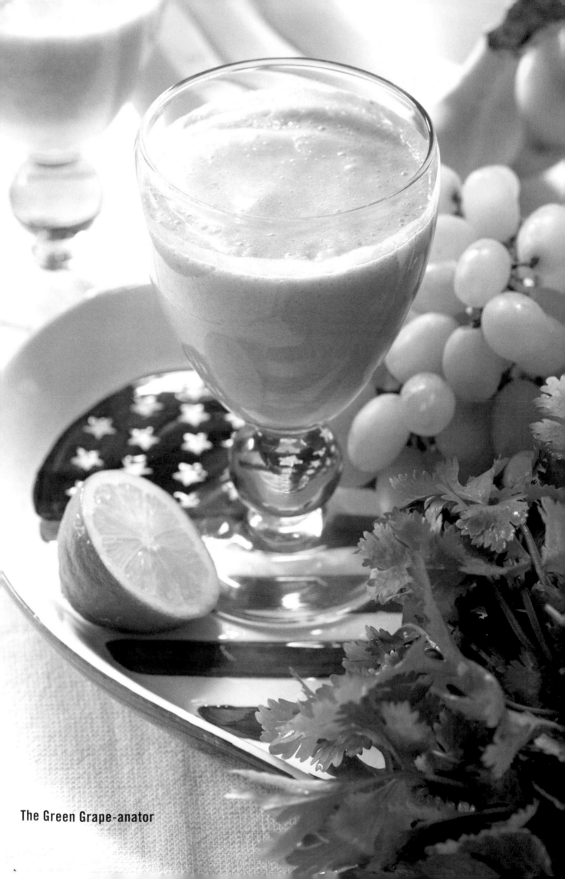

The Green Grape-anator

PEANUT BUTTER AND STRAWBERRY SHAKE

A new twist on an old favorite. Imagine a peanut butter and jelly you can drink. This shake gives you the luxurious flavors of a childhood favorite, as well as the health benefits you want today. Full of protein, antioxidants, and a nice kick of fiber, the taste and nutrient count delivers a satisfying one-two punch. For a thicker shake, increase the ice count by 50 percent.

SERVINGS: 2
SERVING SIZE: 12 OZ

2 cups frozen strawberries (substitute fresh if desired and available)
1 cup of vitamin D-fortified whole milk (or substitute with low-fat or skim milk or unsweetened almond, soy, or coconut milk)
1 ripe medium banana, peeled and sliced
1 tablespoon unsalted organic peanut butter
1 teaspoon organic vanilla protein powder (or substitute organic whey or pea protein powder)
10 small ice cubes

Combine all ingredients in a blender and purée until smooth. Drink and smile!

NUTRITIONAL INFORMATION PER SERVING: 233 cal., 8 g fat, 3 g sat. fat, 35 g carb., 8 g protein, 64 mg sodium, 20 g sugar, 5 g fiber.

VICTORIOUS VANILLA SHAKE

The vanilla shake is as American as apple pie. It conjures up images of hot summer days and parades on Main Street. Ice cream, typically the central ingredient, can be replaced to make this traditional favorite lower in calories but still tasty. A little protein powder helps to make this drink even more filling. Adjust the number of ice cubes based on your desired thickness—the more ice cubes, the thicker the drink. Enjoy this classic at half the calories without losing an ounce of flavor.

SERVINGS: 2
SERVING SIZE: 12 OZ

1½ cups vitamin D-fortified whole milk (or substitute 2 percent reduced-fat milk, or unsweetened almond, soy or coconut milk)
1 ripe small banana, peeled and sliced
2 tablespoons nonfat vanilla yogurt

2 teaspoons raw organic honey
1 teaspoon organic vanilla hemp protein powder (or substitute organic vanilla whey or pea protein powder)
½ teaspoon pure vanilla extract
12 small ice cubes

Combine all ingredients in a blender and purée until smooth. Drink with delight!

NUTRITIONAL INFORMATION PER SERVING: 198 cal., 6 g fat, 4 g sat. fat, 29 g carb., 8 g protein, 23 mg sodium, 23 g sugar, 2 g fiber.

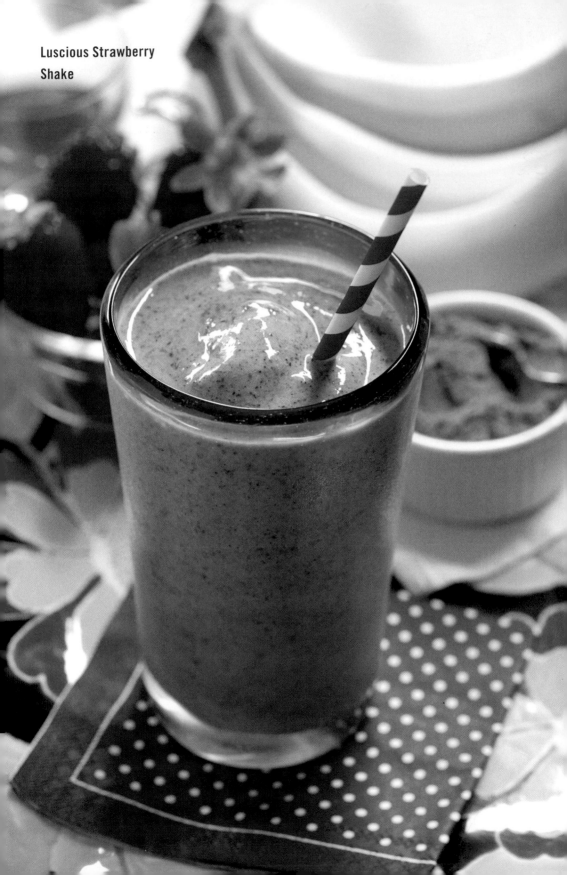

Luscious Strawberry
Shake

LUSCIOUS STRAWBERRY SHAKE

There's nothing like a thick and fruity shake. This strawberry shake delivers great taste with fewer calories. A drink that's sustaining enough to replace a meal, this creamy strawberry shake does not disappoint. A little flaxseed oil adds omega-3 fatty acids, and the flaxseeds themselves add fiber and protein.

SERVINGS: 2
SERVING SIZE: 12 OZ

2½ cups frozen strawberries
1 cup vitamin D-fortified whole milk (or substitute 2 percent reduced-fat milk, or unsweetened almond, soy, or coconut milk)
1 ripe medium banana, peeled and sliced
2 tablespoons organic vanilla hemp protein powder (or substitute organic vanilla whey or pea protein powder)
1 tablespoon ground flaxseed
½ tablespoon unfiltered organic flaxseed oil
1 teaspoon raw organic honey (optional)
12 small ice cubes

Combine all ingredients in a blender and purée until smooth. Enjoy!

NUTRITIONAL INFORMATION PER SERVING: 293 cal., 12 g fat, 3 g sat. fat, 43 g carb., 8 g protein, 66 mg sodium, 24 g sugar, 8 g fiber.

PEANUT BUTTER SWIZZLE SHAKE

The rich flavors of this shake, combined with the creamy texture, let you know right away that you're in store for something special. Bursting with protein, loaded with fiber, long on taste, you get more than your money's worth with this shake. The blueberries add just a hint of sweetness to liven up the flavors as they wash over your tongue. Other drinks that might give you this powerful concentration of nutrients would do so at a much higher calorie count. But the Peanut Butter Swizzle keeps calorie count down and the nutritional value sky-high.

SERVINGS: 2
SERVING SIZE: 12 OZ

1¼ cups whole milk (or substitute 2% reduced-fat milk, unsweetened almond, soy, or coconut milk)
1 cup frozen strawberries
1 banana, peeled and sliced
1 tablespoon unsalted organic peanut butter
1 tablespoon unfiltered organic flaxseed oil
1 teaspoon organic chocolate hemp protein powder (or substitute organic chocolate whey protein powder)
10 small ice cubes

Combine all ingredients in a blender and purée until smooth. Enjoy the rich flavors!

NUTRITIONAL INFORMATION PER SERVING: 289 cal., 16 g fat, 5 g sat. fat, 30 g carb., 8 g protein, 66 mg sodium, 18 g sugar, 4 g fiber.

FEARLESS FILLING FIBROUS SMOOTHIE

Welcome to the king of all fiber drinks. Almost every ingredient in this drink contributes fiber, making 1 serving almost half of your daily recommended fiber intake. The yogurt loads you up on calcium and lots of protein to complement all of the cleansing activities of fiber. Some yogurts actually contain added vitamin D, so for a little bonus, read the nutrition label and opt for one that does. Vitamin D works hand in hand to improve the health of your bones and prevent the all-too-common osteoporosis, a condition in which the bones thin and are at risk for fractures. The other significant feature of this smoothie is that all of the fiber will keep you nice and full for a longer time on fewer calories.

SERVINGS: 2
SERVING SIZE: 12 OZ

1 cup Gala apples, peeled, cored, and sliced
1 cup red Anjou pears, peeled, cored, and sliced
1 cup loosely packed chopped beet greens, stems removed
1 cup loosely packed chopped romaine or green oak leaf lettuce

½ cup nonfat blueberry Greek yogurt
½ cup fresh orange juice
Juice of ½ large lemon
½ teaspoon hemp seeds
6 small ice cubes

Combine the ingredients in a blender and purée until smooth. Drink with gusto!

NUTRITIONAL INFORMATION PER SERVING: 166 cal., 1 g fat, 0 g sat. fat, 35 g carb., 5 g protein, 88 mg sodium, 23 g sugar, 4 g fiber.

BANANA BOAT SHAKE

They don't come as simple as this. The Banana Boat is a wonderful combination of two very different but equally powerful foods. Bananas are a good source of potassium, an essential mineral for maintaining normal blood pressure and heart function. The megadose of potassium in bananas protects the heart and promotes calcium absorption. Drink this before a strenuous workout for an energy punch. It'll sustain your blood sugar and also help prevent pesky muscle cramps.

SERVINGS: 2
SERVING SIZE: 12 OZ

1¼ cups vitamin D-fortified milk (or substitute 2 percent reduced-fat milk; or unsweetened almond, soy, or coconut milk)
1 ripe large banana, peeled and sliced
2 tablespoons old-fashioned rolled oats
1 teaspoon organic vanilla hemp protein powder (or substitute organic vanilla whey or pea protein powder)
1 teaspoon raw organic honey
⅛ teaspoon ground cinnamon
10 small ice cubes

Combine all ingredients in a blender and purée until smooth. Enjoy!

NUTRITIONAL INFORMATION PER SERVING: 190 cal., 5 g fat, 3 g sat. fat, 30 g carb., 7 g protein, 79 mg sodium, 19 g sugar, 3 g fiber.

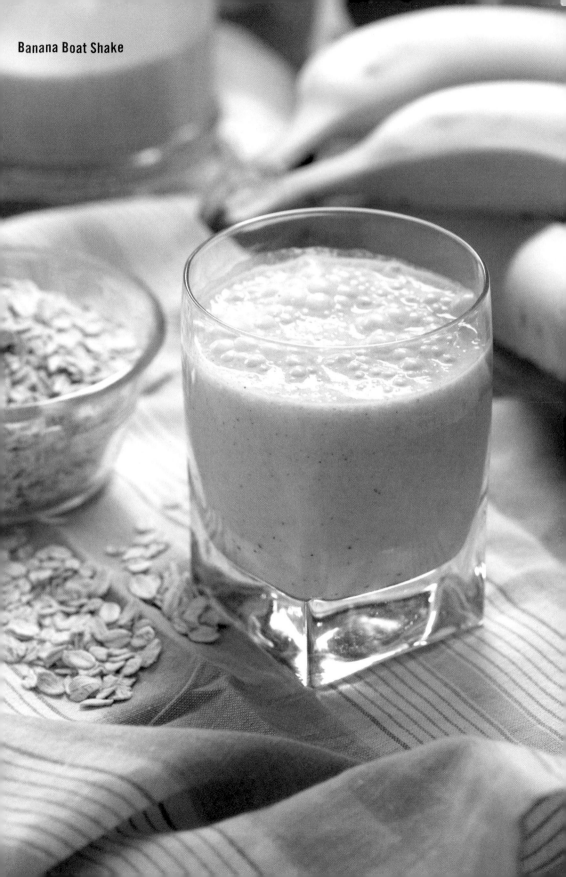

Banana Boat Shake

SUNSHINE BURST SMOOTHIE

A mélange of orange fruits loads up this bright, luxurious, and full-flavored drink with more than just appetizing colors. Peaches originated in China and have been cultivated at least since 1000 BCE. The peach tree is celebrated in Chinese culture as the Tree of Life, where peaches are symbols of immortality and unity. Beyond their beauty and historical significance, they also pack in the nutrition, pumping in fiber as well as vitamins A and C. They are also rich in vital minerals such as potassium, fluoride, and iron. Typically regarded as a summer fruit because their harvest peaks from June to August, frozen peaches allow you to enjoy this wonderful fruit all year round. The oranges nicely complement the peaches, boosting the vitamin C count and mixing in wonderful amounts of some of the B vitamins.

SERVINGS: 2
SERVING SIZE: 12 OZ

2 large oranges, peeled, sliced into sections and seeded
1 cup fresh peach slices (or substitute frozen if fresh are not available)
1 ripe small banana, peeled and sliced
2 tablespoons nonfat vanilla yogurt
½ teaspoon unfiltered organic flaxseed oil
½ small lemon, peeled, sliced into sections, and seeded
8 small ice cubes

Combine the ingredients in a blender and purée until smooth. Drink with gusto!

NUTRITIONAL INFORMATION PER SERVING: 190 cal., 1 g fat, 0 g sat. fat, 46 g carb., 5 g protein, 10 mg sodium, 32 g sugar, 7 g fiber.

PURPLE PINEAPPLE SMOOTHIE

This drink takes two very different fruits and combines them in a surprisingly tasty way. The deep sweetness of the blueberry accents the more concentrated nectar of the pineapple, with both fruits challenged by the relative tartness of the plums. Sporting a low glycemic index (slower rise of blood sugar during digestion) and a low calorie count, plums make a wonderful nutritional addition to this drink. They help increase the absorption of iron into the body, are a good source of vitamin C, and fresh plums contain unique antioxidants called *neochlorogenic* and *chlorogenic acid*, which neutralize dangerous free radicals and prevent cellular damage. This juicy trifecta of fruits doesn't just look tasty, but delivers a heavy uppercut that can knock out potentially bad health.

SERVINGS: 2
SERVING SIZE: 12 OZ

1 cup frozen pineapple chunks
½ cup frozen blueberries
½ cup diced ripe plums
½ cup low-fat plain yogurt
½ cup cold-pressed apple juice
(substitute fresh if available)

¼ cup lightly packed chopped
fresh mint leaves
1 teaspoon unfiltered organic
flaxseed oil

Combine the ingredients in a blender and purée until smooth. Drink with delight!

NUTRITIONAL INFORMATION PER SERVING: 177 cal., 4 g fat, 1 g sat. fat, 34 g carb., 4 g protein, 47 mg sodium, 20 g sugar, 4 g fiber.

WATERMELON EXTRAVAGANZA SMOOTHIE

The light sweetness of watermelon works well with almost anything. It is rather unselfish and allows other flavors to share the stage. Low in calories, but high in vitamins A and C, watermelon is believed by some to contain more of the antioxidant lycopene than any other fruit or vegetable in the world. And don't forget about the folate, magnesium, selenium, choline, and vitamin B6 that it carries along for good measure. The pairing of watermelons and strawberries is definitely a winning combination.

SERVINGS: 2
SERVING SIZE: 12 OZ

2 cups chopped ripe seedless watermelon
1 cup cold-pressed apple juice (substitute fresh if available, or unsweetened coconut water or coconut milk)

1 cup frozen or fresh sliced strawberries
3 tablespoons nonfat strawberry yogurt
1 tablespoon ground flaxseed
1 cup small ice cubes or ½ cup ice chips

Combine the ingredients in a blender and purée until smooth. Revel in the great flavors!

NUTRITIONAL INFORMATION PER SERVING: 165 cal., 2 g fat, 0 g sat. fat, 37 g carb., 3 g protein, 22 mg sodium, 29 g sugar, 5 g fiber.

STRAWBERRY OPENER SMOOTHIE

A great way to start your day is with strawberries and oatmeal. In a rush? No problem—you can put it all in a drink and be on your way. This drink has all that you need in a good breakfast—great taste, enough calories for a burst of energy, ease of preparation, and the phytonutrients that your body craves. Just a quarter cup of oats provides excellent quantities of manganese, phosphorous, copper, vitamin B7, vitamin B1, magnesium, and zinc. As if that weren't enough, this small amount of oats provides 16 percent of your day's recommended fiber and as much as 13 percent of the protein that you need. The strawberries are no slouch either. Not only do they add great taste, but they throw in lots of vitamin C, vitamin B9, potassium, and more fiber. This smoothie is a tremendous start to your day.

SERVINGS: 2
SERVING SIZE: 12 OZ

1½ cups frozen strawberries
1 cup 2 percent reduced-fat milk
   (or substitute unsweetened
   almond, soy, or coconut milk)
1 medium banana, peeled
   and sliced

½ cup old-fashioned rolled oats
4 tablespoons nonfat
   strawberry yogurt
½ teaspoon pure vanilla
   extract

Combine all ingredients in a blender and purée until smooth. Drink and be happy!

NUTRITIONAL INFORMATION PER SERVING: 258 cal., 4 g fat, 2 g sat. fat, 47 g carb., 9 g protein, 73 mg sodium, 23 g sugar, 6 g fiber.

AVARICIOUS AVOCADO SMOOTHIE

Avocados are one of the world's most flexible fruits. Mash them to make great guacamole, chunk them and mix into a tomato salad, or put on a sandwich to add flavor and creamy mouthfeel. You can even put avocado in a smoothie and make use of all of its creamy goodness. Potassium, vitamin B6, vitamin C, and monounsaturated fats are just some of the benefits that avocado brings to the party. Its flavor is full, but also not overbearing, so it serves as a good teammate in this sweet green blend with a kick of lime.

SERVINGS: 2
SERVING SIZE: 12 OZ

1½ cups cold-pressed apple juice (substitute fresh if available)
2 small Bosc or Bartlett pears, peeled, cored, and sliced
½ cup tightly packed curly kale, stems removed
½ ripe avocado, peeled, pitted, and chopped
½ teaspoon pure vanilla extract
1 teaspoon raw organic honey
Juice of ½ small lime
10 small ice cubes

Combine all ingredients in a blender and purée until smooth. Drink and enjoy!

NUTRITIONAL INFORMATION PER SERVING: 298 cal., 7 g fat, 1 g sat. fat, 60 g carb., 3 g protein, 17 mg sodium, 41 g sugar, 11 g fiber.

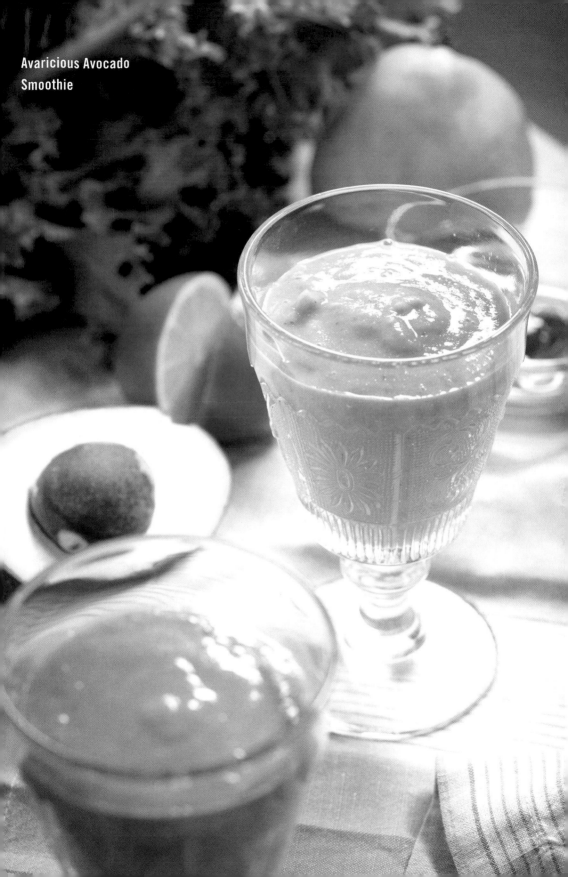

Avaricious Avocado
Smoothie

HONEYDEW ELIXIR SMOOTHIE

Fat-free, cholesterol-free, very low in sodium, low in calories, and dripping with sweetness, the honeydew melon was created to be blended in a smoothie. Although the nutritional value of this melon is often ignored or taken for granted, attention is deserved for its significant amount of vitamin C, as well as important quantities of potassium and vitamin B6. Selecting a ripe melon can make a big difference in the taste, so make sure you search for a melon with a creamy white or pale rind and one that's fragrant before being sliced. Sweet, packed with phytonutrients, and gorgeous in a glass, this smoothie never disappoints.

SERVINGS: 2
SERVING SIZE: 12 OZ

2 cups honeydew melon, peeled, seeded, and sliced

1 cup cold-pressed apple juice (substitute fresh if available, or coconut water)

1 large Granny Smith apple, peeled, cored, and sliced

½ cup tightly packed baby spinach, stems removed

1 small kiwi, peeled and sliced

Juice of ½ large lemon

1 tablespoon unfiltered organic flaxseed oil

Combine all ingredients in a blender and purée until smooth. Have a good time!

NUTRITIONAL INFORMATION PER SERVING: 251 cal., 7 g fat, 1 g sat. fat, 48 g carb., 2 g protein, 41 mg sodium, 40 g sugar, 3 g fiber.

THE ARISTOCRAT

Cucumber sandwiches conjure images of sumptuous sitting rooms and sterling tea services shining under crystal chandeliers. Crunchy, light, and easily adaptable, cucumbers are enjoyable in everything from salads to sandwiches to chilled water. Cucumbers might be low in calories, but they are high in the phytonutrients of cucurbitacins, lignans, and flavonoids, which have antioxidant, antiinflammatory, and anticancer benefits. Throw in the fiber from pears and kale and a little kick of ginger, and the cucumber becomes a true delight for the masses.

1½ cups unsweetened coconut milk (or substitute unsweetened almond or soy milk)
2 small Bartlett pears, peeled, cored, and sliced
½ cup loosely packed curly kale, stems removed
One 6-inch piece cucumber, peeled and sliced (optional to remove seeds)
⅛ teaspoon peeled and grated ginger
10 small ice cubes

Combine all ingredients in a blender and purée until smooth. Enjoy every drop!

NUTRITIONAL INFORMATION PER SERVING: 192 cal., 6 g fat, 5 g sat. fat, 41 g carb., 2 g protein, 86 mg sodium, 21 g sugar, 7 g fiber.

CHICAGO SMOOTHIE

The Windy City built on the shores of Lake Michigan is famous for its deep-dish pizza, Polish sausages, and Italian beef. But Chicagoans also know a good smoothie when they drink one. The combination of blueberries, grapes, cherries, and Swiss chard creates a thrilling flavor that could be enjoyed from the South Side marina all the way to the sands of Oak Street Beach to the north. A sweet combination of fiber, antioxidants, and omega-3 fatty acids provides a filling drink equally enjoyable during the bone-chilling long winters or the sweltering heat of a typical July's Taste of Chicago.

SERVINGS: 2
SERVING SIZE: 12 OZ

1 cup frozen blueberries
1 cup black seedless grapes, frozen
1 cup frozen pitted cherries (substitute fresh if available)
1 cup tightly packed chopped Swiss chard, stems removed
1 cup cold-pressed apple juice (substitute fresh if available)
1 ripe small banana, peeled and sliced
2 tablespoons nonfat vanilla yogurt
1 tablespoon unfiltered organic flaxseed oil
8 small ice cubes

Combine all ingredients in a blender and purée until smooth. Have a blast!

NUTRITIONAL INFORMATION PER SERVING: 259 cal., 18 g fat, 1 g sat. fat, 48 g carb., 4 g protein, 50 mg sodium, 35 g sugar, 7 g fiber.

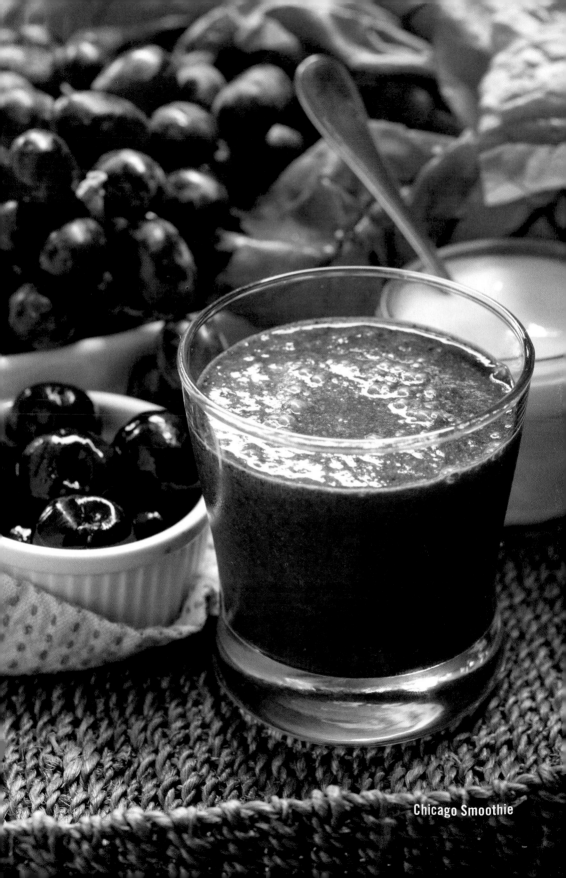

Chicago Smoothie

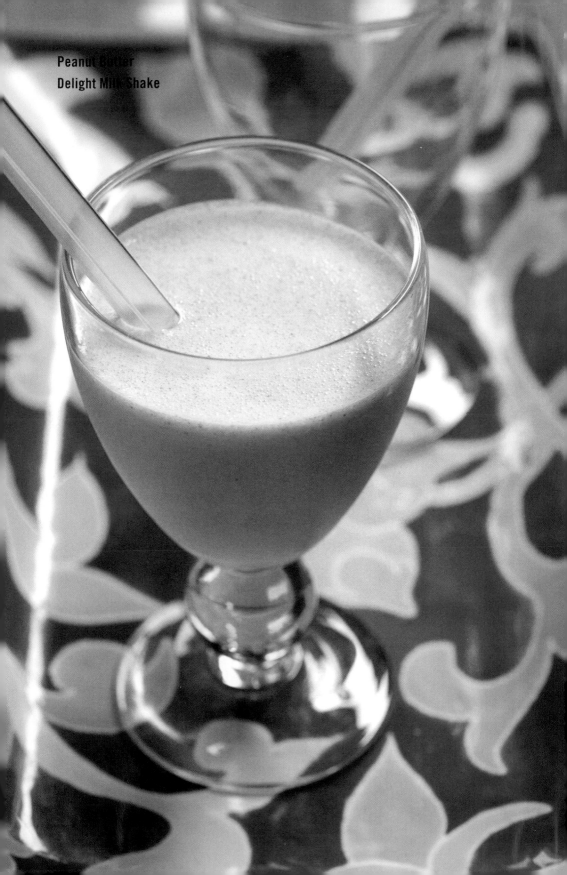

Peanut Butter
Delight Milk Shake

PEANUT BUTTER DELIGHT MILK SHAKE

The combination of peanut butter, banana, and oats may not be what first comes to mind when you think of a great shake, but this drink delivers on many levels. Almost half of your day's requirement of protein is pleasantly packed in this creamy mixture. Then you get a tremendous dose of cleansing fiber—as much as 50 percent of your day's recommended daily intake. And the rich taste of peanut butter sliding over the distinctive flavor of oats is sweetened by the banana that holds it all together. The Peanut Butter Delight not only keeps hunger away but loads you up on a host of lively nutrients while doing so.

SERVINGS: 2
SERVING SIZE: 12 OZ

1¼ cup cold 2% vitamin D-fortified milk (or substitute whole milk for a thicker shake; or unsweetened, almond, soy, or coconut milk)	1 tablespoon unfiltered organic flaxseed oil
1 ripe large banana, peeled and sliced	1 tablespoon unsalted organic peanut butter
2½ tablespoons old-fashioned rolled oats	1 teaspoon raw organic honey
	10 small ice cubes

Combine all ingredients in a blender and purée until smooth. Drink and enjoy!

NUTRITIONAL INFORMATION PER SERVING: 298 cal., 18 g fat, 3 g sat. fat, 34 g carb., 9 g protein, 81 mg sodium, 21 g sugar, 3 g fiber.

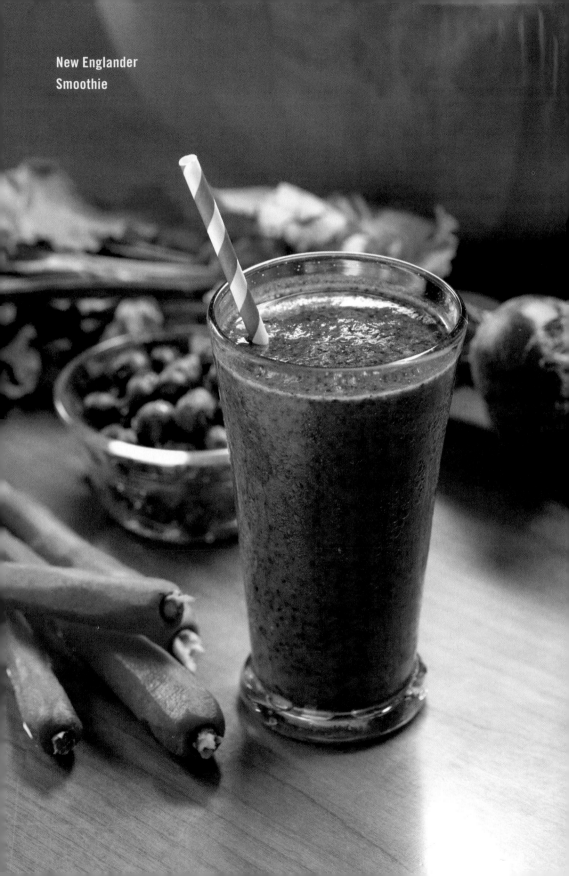

New Englander
Smoothie

NEW ENGLANDER SMOOTHIE

Dark purple beets are a good match for the hardy New England earth and its chilled weather. Beets, in fact, are one of a relatively few vegetables that can be planted in the fall and grow in cold weather. The red color is also a giveaway for all of the phytonutrients it contains. Beets are a unique source of betalains, specifically betanin and vulgaxanthin, compounds that have been shown to provide antioxidant, antiinflammatory, and detoxification support. Although there are other foods that contain betalains, beets have them in great concentration in their peel and flesh. These root vegetables also supply appreciable amounts of folate, manganese, potassium, copper, fiber, magnesium, phosphorous, vitamin C, and iron. With an earthy taste and naturally sweet undertones, beets are a surprisingly capable ingredient in a full-flavored smoothie.

SERVINGS: 2
SERVING SIZE: 12 OZ

1½ cups cold-pressed apple juice
   (substitute fresh if available)
1 cup frozen blueberries
1 medium beet, chopped

¼ cup peeled and chopped carrots
1 tablespoon unfiltered organic
   flaxseed oil
10 small ice cubes

Combine all ingredients in a blender and purée until smooth. Enjoy greatly!

NUTRITIONAL INFORMATION PER SERVING: 209 cal., 8 g fat, 1 g sat. fat, 37 g carb., 1 g protein, 47 mg sodium, 30 g sugar, 5 g fiber.

THE NEW YORKER

New York City is believed to have gotten its nickname from two African-American stable hands at the famed New Orleans Fair Grounds. They imagined that *The Big Apple* was an apt name for one of the city's major horse-racing prizes. The apple remains one of the most popular fruits in the world. Its fiber, vitamin C, antioxidants, and polyphenols help prevent blood sugar spikes. Pair apples with strawberries; a pinch of ginger; and some spinach for vitamins A and K, folate, and fiber, and you have a prize-winning smoothie.

SERVINGS: 2
SERVING SIZE: 12 OZ

1½ cups unsweetened chilled coconut water
2 large Gala or Honeycrip apples, peeled, cored, and sliced
1 cup frozen strawberry slices (substitute with fresh if desired)

½ cup loosely packed baby spinach, stems removed
⅛ teaspoon ground ginger (substitute with fresh grated ginger if desired)
10 small ice cubes

Combine all ingredients in a blender and purée until smooth. Drink and be merry!

NUTRITIONAL INFORMATION PER SERVING: 178 cal., 0 g fat, 0 g sat. fat, 46 g carb., 1 g protein, 98 mg sodium, 34 g sugar, 7 g fiber.

HONEY BALSAMIC VINAIGRETTE

SERVING SIZE: 2 TABLESPOONS

⅛ cup extra-virgin olive oil
2 tablespoons white balsamic
   vinegar
1 tablespoon raw organic honey

1 teaspoon Dijon mustard
½ teaspoon dried basil
Salt and black pepper

In a small bowl, whisk together the olive oil, vinegar, honey, mustard, and dried basil. Season with salt and pepper to taste.

NUTRITIONAL INFORMATION PER SERVING: 68 cal., 14 g fat, 2 g sat. fat, 2.5 g carb., 0 g protein, 108 mg sodium, 2.5 g sugar, 0 g fiber.

ORANGE RASPBERRY VINAIGRETTE

½ cup freshly squeezed orange
  juice, no added sugars
¼ cup raspberry white balsamic
  vinegar
⅛ cup extra-virgin olive oil
1 teaspoon chopped fresh cilantro
  leaves
Salt and black pepper

In a small bowl, whisk together the orange juice, vinegar, olive oil, and cilantro. Season with salt and pepper to taste.

NUTRITIONAL INFORMATION PER SERVING: 69 cal., 7 g fat, 2 g sat. fat, 6 g carb., .5 g protein, 78 mg sodium, 4.5 g sugar, 0 g fiber.

INDEX

To order SHRED POP all natural popcorn, go to www.shredlife.com.